A GENERAL INTRODUCTION TO TRADITIONAL CHINESE MEDICINE

A GENERAL INTRODUCTION TO TRADITIONAL CHINESE MEDICINE

Edited by

Men Jiuzhang

Guo Lei

Science Press

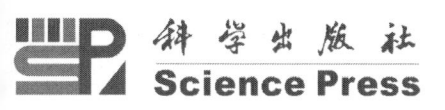

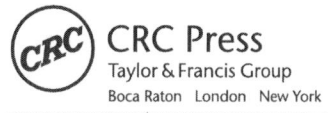

CRC Press
Taylor & Francis Group
Boca Raton London New York

CRC Press is an imprint of the
Taylor & Francis Group, an **informa** business

CRC Press
Taylor & Francis Group
6000 Broken Sound Parkway NW, Suite 300
Boca Raton, FL 33487-2742

© 2010 by Science Press
CRC Press is an imprint of Taylor & Francis Group, an Informa business

No claim to original U.S. Government works

10 9 8 7 6 5 4 3 2 1

International Standard Book Number: 978-1-4200-9044-4 (Hardback)

This book contains information obtained from authentic and highly regarded sources. Reasonable efforts have been made to publish reliable data and information, but the author and publisher cannot assume responsibility for the validity of all materials or the consequences of their use. The authors and publishers have attempted to trace the copyright holders of all material reproduced in this publication and apologize to copyright holders if permission to publish in this form has not been obtained. If any copyright material has not been acknowledged please write and let us know so we may rectify in any future reprint.

Except as permitted under U.S. Copyright Law, no part of this book may be reprinted, reproduced, transmitted, or utilized in any form by any electronic, mechanical, or other means, now known or hereafter invented, including photocopying, microfilming, and recording, or in any information storage or retrieval system, without written permission from the publishers.

For permission to photocopy or use material electronically from this work, please access www.copyright.com (http://www.copyright.com/) or contact the Copyright Clearance Center, Inc. (CCC), 222 Rosewood Drive, Danvers, MA 01923, 978-750-8400. CCC is a not-for-profit organization that provides licenses and registration for a variety of users. For organizations that have been granted a photocopy license by the CCC, a separate system of payment has been arranged.

Trademark Notice: Product or corporate names may be trademarks or registered trademarks, and are used only for identification and explanation without intent to infringe.

Library of Congress Cataloging-in-Publication Data

Men, Jiuzhang.
　A general introduction to traditional Chinese medicine / Men Jiuzhang and Guo Lei.
　　p. ; cm.
　Includes bibliographical references and index.
　ISBN 978-1-4200-9044-4 (hardcover : alk. paper)
　1. Medicine, Chinese. I. Guo, Lei, 1968- II. Title.
　[DNLM: 1. Medicine, Chinese Traditional. WB 55.C4 M488g 2010]

R601.M37 2010
616'.09--dc22
　　　　　　　　　　　　　　　　　　　　　　　　　　　　　　　　　　　　　　2009016718

Visit the Taylor & Francis Web site at
http://www.taylorandfrancis.com

and the CRC Press Web site at
http://www.crcpress.com

Contents

Preface

Chapter 1 Introduction 1
- 1.1 Establishment and Development of TCM's Academic System 1
  - 1.1.1 Primitive Society 1
  - 1.1.2 The Shang Dynasty (1600–1046 B.C.) 2
  - 1.1.3 The Zhou Dynasty (1046–256 B.C.) and the Spring and Autumn Period (770–476 B.C.) 2
  - 1.1.4 The Qin and the Han Dynasties (221 B.C.–220 A.D.) 3
  - 1.1.5 From the Sui Dynasty to the Yuan Dynasty (581–1368 A.D.) 4
  - 1.1.6 The Ming (1368–1644 A.D.) and Qing Dynasties (1644–1911 A.D.) 5
- 1.2 Great Historical Achievements of Early TCM 5
  - 1.2.1 The Qin and Han Dynasties (221 B.C.–220 A.D.) 5
  - 1.2.2 The Jin Dynasty (265–420 A.D.) 6
  - 1.2.3 The Tang, Song, and Yuan Dynasties (618–1368 A.D.) 7
  - 1.2.4 The Ming and Qing Dynasties (1368–1911 A.D.) 8
- 1.3 Basic Theoretical Views of TCM 8
  - 1.3.1 The Outlook of Man and Nature 9
  - 1.3.2 TCM's Physiological and Pathological Outlooks 11
  - 1.3.3 TCM's Outlook on Health Maintenance and Treatment 13

Chapter 2 Theoretical System of TCM: Formation and Characters 17
- 2.1 The Formation of the Theoretical System of TCM 17
  - 2.1.1 The Promotion of Social Culture 17
  - 2.1.2 Experiential Accumulation 18
  - 2.1.3 The Observation of Life Phenomena 18
  - 2.1.4 The Penetration of Philosophical Ideas 19
- 2.2 The Disciplinary Properties of TCM 20
  - 2.2.1 Multidisciplinary Properties: Natural Science, Humanistic-Social Science, and Philosophy 21
  - 2.2.2 TCM: Both Basic and Applied Disciplines 22

Chapter 3 Clinical System of TCM: Formation and Development 27
- 3.1 Accumulation of Clinical Experiences 27
  - 3.1.1 Primitive Cognition of Disease 27
  - 3.1.2 From Witches' Practice to Medical Treatment 28
  - 3.1.3 Medication Development: From Single-Symptom-and-Single-Medicine-Based Medication to Compound-Symptom-and-Prescription-Based Medication 28
- 3.2 Exploration of Disease's Cause and Law 29
  - 3.2.1 *The Classic of Internal Medicine* and *The Classic of Medical Problems*: Explorations of the Cause and Law of Disease 29
  - 3.2.2 *The Classic of Meteria Medica*: Pharmacological Development 30
- 3.3 Preliminary Establishment of TSD 30
- 3.4 Accumulation of Therapeutic Experiences 33
  - 3.4.1 Furthering Cognition of Disease 34
  - 3.4.2 Improving Therapeutic Understanding 34

3.5 Theory Inheritance and Practice Standardization 35
3.6 Complete Summary of Clinical Experiences and the Perfection of the
    TSD Model 36

Chapter 4 Basic Features of TCM 37
  4.1 The Concept of Holism 38
    4.1.1 The Human Body: An Organic Integrity 38
    4.1.2 The Unity of Man and Nature 43
  4.2 Treatment Based on Syndrome Differentiation (TSD) 46
    4.2.1 Specific Contents of TSD 47
    4.2.2 Relationship between Syndrome Differentiation and Treatment 51
    4.2.3 The Principles of TSD 51
    4.2.4 Superiority of TSD 54

Chapter 5 Philosophical Foundation of TCM 55
  5.1 The Theory of Primordial *Qi* 56
    5.1.1 The Formation and Development of the Theory of Primordial *Qi* 56
    5.1.2 The Basic Contents of the Theory of Primordial *Qi* 56
    5.1.3 The Application of the Theory of Primordial *Qi* in TCM 58
  5.2 The Theory of *Yin-yang* 59
    5.2.1 The Origin and Formation of the *Yin-yang* Theory 60
    5.2.2 The Basic Concept of *Yin-yang* 61
    5.2.3 Basic Contents of *Yin-yang* Theory 63
    5.2.4 The Application of *Yin-yang* Theory in TCM 68
  5.3 The Theory of Five Elements 77
    5.3.1 The Formation and Development of the Theory of Five Elements 77
    5.3.2 The Characteristics of Five Elements 78
    5.3.3 Categorization and Deduction of Things in Terms of Five Elements .. 79
    5.3.4 Fundamental Contents of the Theory of Five Elements 82
    5.3.5 Application of the Theory of Five Elements in TCM 87
  5.4 Interrelationships among Theories of Primordial *Qi*, *Yin-yang*, and
      Five Elements 98

Chapter 6 Model, Method, and Architecture of TCM 99
  6.1 The Model of TCM 99
    6.1.1 Preliminary Establishment of the Bio-psycho-social-medical Model ... 99
    6.1.2 TCM's Peculiar Model and Its Principle 102
  6.2 The Method of TCM 103
    6.2.1 General Philosophical Methods of TCM 103
    6.2.2 Specific Research Methods of TCM 104
  6.3 The Architecture of TCM 107
    6.3.1 A Summary of the Fundamental Theories of TCM 108
    6.3.2 A Summary of the Clinical System 110

Main References 113
Endnotes 115
Glossary 121
Subject Index 127
Title Index 131
Name Index 133

Preface

A General Introduction to Traditional Chinese Medicine is an introductory book on Traditional Chinese Medicine (TCM). It attempts to guide readers to learn TCM's academic thoughts, theoretical system, and clinical practice. The book is trying to provide beginners with TCM's peculiar way of thinking, more than 2,000 years' history, and TCM's philosophy-based theoretical system.

The book covers:
- Establishment and characteristics of TCM's theoretical system.
- Establishment and development of TCM's clinical system.
- Basic features of TCM.
- TCM's philosophical bases: primordial *qi*, *yin-yang*, and Five Elements, and
- TCM's medical model, method, and architecture.

The book has been carefully designed to be as accessible as possible, with

- **Objectives & Requirements** and **Key Concepts** are at the beginning of every chapter to enable readers to understand the core and the outline of the chapter.
- **Endnotes**, not only as one essential part of references for readers to learn more about TCM, but also as a guide for foreign readers to learn some cultural and historical information peculiar to China.
- **Glossary** for readers to understand more specific information about TCM and Chinese culture.

We would like to acknowledge a few Chinese famous professors like professor He Yuming from Shanghai University of TCM and Zhang Zhenyu from Shandong University of TCM for their academic enlightenment; our grateful thanks also go to colleagues and friends who share their expertise by contributing materials, reading drafts, and fruitful conversation; we also owe our abundant thanks to the translators of the book, Li Xia from Shanxi University of TCM, and Chai Gaiying and Curtis Evans from Zhejiang Gongshang University.

We hope that you will find useful the design, the content, and the support the book will give to your research and practice.

Men Jiuzhang & Guo Lei
Editors

CHAPTER 1

Introduction

Objectives & Requirements

1. Important contents of the initial theoretical system of Traditional Chinese Medicine (TCM).
2. Historical development of TCM.
3. Historical achievements of TCM.
4. Basic views of TCM.

Key Concepts

Traditional Chinese Medicine (TCM), as a part of medicine in the world, is a great treasure-house. Its unique theoretical system was preliminarily established in the Western Han dynasty (206 B.C.–25 A.D.) under the influence of ancient materialism and dialectics. Its development is closely related to two thousand years of Chinese society, culture, and philosophy, as well as its science and technology. It is not only the summarization of a rich medical practice, but also the crystallization of ancient Chinese wisdom. This chapter will introduce the historical development, the achievements, and the academic characteristics of TCM.

Early in the Spring and Autumn Period (722–481 B.C.) and the Warring States Period (475–221 B.C.), TCM, as a systematic and an independent disciplinary system, had already laid its theoretical and clinical foundations. Its unique medical method and rich practical experience not only make a great contribution to the healthcare and the prosperity of China, but also have a profound influence on the world medical system. Especially in the 21st century, through the cultural exchange between the East and the West, TCM has been increasingly recognized thanks to its curative effect. To understand TCM systematically, one has to have a good command of its historical and cultural background, its systematic features, the scientific nature of its practice, and the special cultural form of its theoretical expression.

1.1 Establishment and Development of TCM's Academic System

TCM is an academic system about human physiology and pathology, as well as the diagnosis and treatment of diseases. Its establishment is based on thousands of years of experience of Chinese medicine, prescription, principle, and reflection on the relationship between man and nature.

1.1.1 Primitive Society

It is generally believed that Chinese medicine started from Shennong[1] who tasted hundreds of herbs, among which, according to *Huainan Tzu*,[2] about seventy kinds are poisonous. He warned people not to try them. Such a record vividly reflects how the ancient Chinese learned about medicine (including plants, animals, and minerals) and accumulated pharmacological experiences.

Chinese medical techniques were attempted in primitive society. The famous TCM technique of acupuncture was originated from the stone-needle practice of the Neolithic Age. Ancient Chinese used a kind of sharp stone to break abscesses and discharge blood and pus.

Such a tool is the predecessor of today's knife-like needle used in acupuncture. The effect of the stone-needle practice has been recorded in the ancient books like *Plain Questions*.[3] It is said that "the large carbuncle disease spread in the east and was cured with stone needles" (*Plain Questions, XII*). The primitive tools of acupuncture such as stone needles, bone needles, and bamboo needles gradually developed into cupreous and golden needles, and eventually into today's stainless steel and silver needles.

Another important TCM technique of moxibustion was also used by primitive people to treat diseases. Specifically, they warmed a certain part of the human body by burning, fumigating, or ironing with ignited materials like moxa. The invention of such a method, as *Plain Questions* states, is closely related to the cold living conditions in North China.

1.1.2 The Shang Dynasty (1600–1046 B.C.)

The Shang dynasty, a period with a flourishing brewing industry, introduced wine to the medical field. Wine, a stimulant (in a small amount) and an anesthetic (in a large amount), was found effective in promoting blood circulation and enhancing the curative effects of medications. At that time, this kind of aromatic medicated liquid was also used as a sort of solvent. *The Classic of Internal Medicine*[4] points out that decoction and wine are used to prevent and treat exogenous diseases, and *History of the Later Han Dynasty*[5] names wine as the king of medications, for wine is not only a medicine itself but also can enhance the effectiveness of other medications. The ancient Chinese character "醫 (medicine)" is made of the components "医" (medicine), "殳" (work), and "酉 (wine)," which proves the critical role of wine in the medical practice in ancient China.

Decoction is recorded to have been invented by Yi Yin, a physician who excelled cooking in the early Shang dynasty. According to *The Records of the Historian*,[6] just like cooking, Yi Yin made liquid medicine by decocting various crude drugs with water. The invention of decoction can be said to symbolize the birth of prescriptions.

1.1.3 The Zhou Dynasty (1046–256 B.C.) and the Spring and Autumn Period (770–476 B.C.)

From the founding of the Western Zhou dynasty in 1046 B.C. to the birth of the Spring and Autumn Period in 770 B.C., the ancient Chinese learned more about poisonous herbs such as *Radix Aconiti*, and *Flos Genkwa*, as well as poisonous minerals such as aluminite. According to the record, poison began to be used to harm others early in the eighth 8th B.C.

The earliest work that records the medicinal herbs extant in China is *The Book of Songs*[7] written in the Spring and Autumn Period. In this book, more than fifty kinds of plant medicines are recorded, such as *Semen Plantaginis*, *Rhizoma Alismatis*, *Radix Puerariae*, *Radix Cynanchi Atrati*, *Radix Glycyrrhizae*, and *Radix Scutellariae*. For certain herbs, their gathering, habitat, and edible effects were concisely described in the book. For example, the verses of "picking melons in July" and "plucking gourds in August" indicate the seasons of gathering; the line "*Herba Leonuri* is in the valley" shows the habitat of herbs; and the line "*Semen Plantaginis* is good for procreation" is a description of its curative effect.

More records about Chinese medicine can be found in the famous book *The Classic of Mountains and Rivers*,[8] which includes 126 types of medications involving sixty-seven kinds of animal drugs, fifty-two kinds of herbal medicines, three kinds of mineral medicines, one kind of aqueous medicine, and three kinds of others that are unknown. Although, like *The Book of Songs*, it is not a specialized medicinal book, it clearly records the habitat, function, and curative effect of medications. For instance, "scrofula can be cured with vanilla" and "scabies can be cured by washing the affected part with herbs of *Asclepiadoideae*."

In addition, a medical system was also formed in the Zhou dynasty. Royal doctors were divided into dietitians, physicians, surgeons, and veterinarians. A set of medical examining and assessing systems as well as a medical service system were established. They also attached due importance to medical records and reports of the cause of death. All of these are of significance in medical history.

1.1.4 The Qin and the Han Dynasties (221 B.C.–220 A.D.)

The Chinese medical systems were initially formed in the Qin and Han dynasties (221 B.C.–220 A.D.). The landmarks are *The Classic of Internal Medicine* and *The Treatise on Exogenous Febrile Diseases and Miscellaneous Diseases*.[9] The former laid an important foundation for TCM's theoretical system with theories like holism, *yin and yang*, Five Elements, etc., and the latter made great contributions to TCM's clinical system, including numerable prescriptions and the establishment of Treatment Based on Syndrome Differentiation (TSD).

1.1.4.1 The Establishment of the Theoretical System of TCM: *The Classic of Internal Medicine*

The publication of *The Classic of Internal Medicine* symbolizes the TCM's evolvement from simple experience accumulation into systemic theoretical summarization and marks the preliminary formation of its theoretical system. The book, produced by many physicians from the Warring States Period to the Qin and the Han dynasties, laid a theoretical foundation for TCM with its concept of holism; the concept of contradictions; the theory of *zang-fu* organs, meridians, and collaterals; the theory of etiology and pathogenesis; the theory of health maintenance and disease prevention; and the principles of diagnosis and treatment. Its achievements can be summarized in the following aspects.

First, *The Classic of Internal Medicine* emphasizes the concept of holism, which not only refers to the integrity of the human body itself, but also the unity of man and nature. As an organic integrity, parts of the human body are inseparable in structure, coordinating in physiology, and mutually influential in pathology. Meanwhile, the human body corresponds with nature in that human beings try to adapt themselves to the natural conditions like the four seasons and geographical environment to maintain their normal vital activities, which is called "correspondence between man and nature."

Second, the book takes the doctrines of *yin-yang* and Five Elements as its philosophical foundation to explain the physiology and pathology of the human body. And they are also the bases of the syndrome differentiation and treatment.

Third, it generalizes another component essential to TCM's theoretical system, the theory of *zang-fu* organs, meridians, and collaterals. It mainly studies the physiological functions and pathological changes of *zang-fu* organs, twelve meridians, and the eight extraordinary meridians, as well as their mutual relations.

Fourth, in the analysis of etiology and pathogenesis, it attaches much importance to the mental and social factors in addition to pathogenic factors. Its rational statements about medical psychology, medical sociology, and healthcare are extremely important in the history of world medicine.

Fifth, the book pays great attention to disease prevention, and its viewpoints of "treating disease before its onset," "giving prevention the priority," and "observing the development of disease from the inconspicuous clinical manifestations," still have a profound significance today.

As a comprehensive medical work of early China, *The Classic of Internal Medicine* greatly influences the world of medicine today. It is a required textbook for medicos in Japan and

Korea, a required reference book for acupuncturists in foreign academic institutes, and has been partially translated into English, German, French, and a number of other languages.

1.1.4.2 The Establishment of the Clinical System of TCM: The Treatise on Exogenous Febrile Diseases and Miscellaneous Diseases

The Treatise on Exogenous Febrile Diseases and Miscellaneous Diseases written by Zhang Zhongjing in the Eastern Han dynasty (25–200 A.D.) established the standards for the diagnosis and treatment of fevers and miscellaneous diseases. It has been prevalent for 1,700 years, because of its rich prescriptions and TSD principles. The book has been popular also in foreign countries since the Tang and Song dynasties; many Japanese professionals not only adopted its prescriptions in treatment, but also made patent medicines according to its prescriptions.

TSD means to decide the therapeutic methods according to the result of syndrome differentiation. Namely, based on the eight diagnostic principles (i.e., *yin*, *yang*, exterior, interior, cold, heat, asthenia, and excess) and the four diagnostic methods (i.e., inspection, auscultation and olfaction, interrogation, and pulse taking and palpation), the doctor analyzes the clinical data to determine the location, cause, and nature of a patient's disease and achieve the diagnosis of a syndrome. The physician finally decides the appropriate basic therapeutic methods (diaphoresis, emesis, purgation, regulating therapy, warming therapy, cooling therapy, supplementing, or resolving therapy). Zhang Zhongjing came up with the theory of the Six Meridians to differentiate exogenous febrile diseases and the theory of *zang-fu* organs to distinguish miscellaneous diseases. As a comprehensive generalization of medical theories, principles, prescriptions, and herbs of TCM, *The Treatise on Exogenous Febrile Diseases and Miscellaneous Diseases* laid a solid foundation for the development of Chinese clinical medicine, encompassing the whole process from diagnosis to treatment.

1.1.5 From the Sui Dynasty to the Yuan Dynasty (581–1368 A.D.)

With the publication of *The Classic of Internal Medicine*, *The Treatise on Exogenous Febrile Diseases and Miscellaneous Diseases*, *The Classic of Medical Problems*,[10] and *The Classic of Materia Medica*,[11] the ancient Chinese medicine and pharmacology were comprehensively summarized. From then on, TCM has been further developed from different perspectives. For example, in the Sui dynasty (581–618 A.D.), Chao Yuanfang compiled *The General Treatise on the Etiology and Symptomatology of Diseases*,[12] the first monograph about etiology, pathogenesis, and symptomatology. In the Song dynasty (960–1279 A.D.), Qian Yi put forward syndrome differentiation of viscera for the first time in his *Therapeusis of Pediatric Diseases*,[13] and Chen Wuze brought forward the famous theory of "Three Types of Etiologic Factors" in *Prescriptions Assigned to the Three Categories of Pathogenic Factors of Diseases*.[14] In the Jin and Yuan dynasties (1115–1368 A.D.), various schools of medicine appeared, represented by the four great physicians in the Jin and Yuan dynasties, Liu Wansu, Zhang Congzheng, Li Gao, and Zhu Zhenheng. Liu Wansu, the founder of "The Cold School of Medicine," believed that excessive heat was the main cause of diseases, which should be dealt with medicines of a cold nature. The theory had much influence on the School of Epidemic Febrile Diseases in the Ming and Qing dynasties. Zhang Congzheng, the initiator of "The Purgation School," held that all diseases were caused by exogenous pathogenic factors, which should be driven out by drastic drugs like diaphoretics, emetics, and purgatives. Li Gao, the father of "The School for Strengthening the Spleen and Stomach," maintained that the internal impairment of spleen and stomach would bring about various diseases and therefore the most important thing in clinical treatment should be to regulate the spleen and stomach and to nourish the original *qi*. Zhu Zhenheng, the founder of "The Yin-Nourishing School," proposed that "*yang* is always in excess while *yin* is frequently deficient" and therefore the best therapeutic method should be to nourish *yin* and purge *fire*. In the Ming dynasty, Zhao Xianke and Zhang Jiebin put forward the theory of "life gate," which was the new manifestation of *zang-xiang* theory in TCM. Though these schools are quite different from each other, their propositions have enriched TCM from different perspectives.

1.1.6 The Ming (1368–1644 A.D.) and Qing Dynasties (1644–1911 A.D.)

In the Ming and Qing dynasties, based on the theories of *The Classic of Internal Medicine*, *The Classic of Medical Problems*, and *The Treatise on Exogenous Febrile Diseases and Miscellaneous Diseases*, the research on seasonal febrile diseases gradually evolved into an independent discipline. Wu Youke (1582–1652) put forward the theory of pestilential factors, which in his opinion were not six exogenous pathogenic factors (wind, cold, summer-heat, dampness, dryness, and heat), but a special pathogenic factor in the natural world, which invades the human body from the mouth and nose rather than through the skin. In the Qing dynasty, Ye Gui and Wu Tang established a complete theoretical system of seasonal febrile diseases with the scheme of four-level syndromes (defensive, *qi*, nutrient, and blood) differentiation and that of the *"triple energizer"* at its core. In addition, in the Qing dynasty, Wang Qingren conducted research on anatomy and compiled *Corrections of the Errors in Medical Works*,[15] rectifying the mistakes about the anatomy of the human body in ancient medical books and developing the theory of the pathogenesis due to blood stagnation.

Since the foundation of the People's Republic of China in 1949, with advanced science and technology, TCM has made outstanding progress in modernizing its therapeutic system from both the perspectives of traditional and modern medicine.

1.2 Great Historical Achievements of Early TCM

TCM, as an important component of traditional Chinese culture, is a great treasure. It not only makes great contributions to the prosperity of China, but also occupies an extremely brilliant position in the history of world medicine.

1.2.1 The Qin and Han Dynasties (221 B.C.–220 A.D.)

The Classic of Internal Medicine written in the Qin and Han dynasties (221 B.C.–220 A.D.) has the earliest cognition of human reproduction, physiological characteristics, physique classification (in terms of individual figure and temperament), the physiological, psychological, and pathological description of various groups of people, anatomic knowledge, as well as the structures and functions of viscera and tissues.

The book also explores the relation between heart and blood circulation. Namely, nutrients from food and drink digested and absorbed by the digestive system goes to the liver, heart, lungs, and then back to the heart again, and afterward they are transported to the whole body. The pulsating blood vessel is an "artery." These understandings about blood circulation are 1,000 years earlier than most of those in western medicine. The similar recognitions were acquired by Claudius Galen in Ancient Rome in the 2nd century, Michael Servetus in Spain in the 16th century, and William Harvey in England in 17th century.

The Classic of Materia Medica, finished in the Eastern Han dynasty (25–220 A.D.), is the earliest classic of pharmacology. Some 365 kinds of medicinal herbs are recorded and a large majority of these have been proven clinically effective. For example, *Herba Ephedrae* can relieve asthma, *Radix Dichroae* can prevent malaria, *Rhizoma Coptidis* can stop dysentery, *Pedicellus Melo Fructus* can induce vomiting, *Sargassum* can cure goiter, *Poria* can induce diuresis, *Radix Scutellariae* can clear heat, and *Omphalia* can kill intestinal parasites. These are great discoveries in world medical history.

In addition, Zhang Zhongjing, an influential physician in the late Eastern Han dynasty, advocated the combination of disease differentiation and syndrome differentiation, and made a detailed exploration into the diagnosis and treatment of jaundice, edema, stroke, amenorrhea, morning sickness, and postpartum diseases. Based on them, he made the first theoretical generalization of prescriptions. His medical work *The Treatise on Exogenous Febrile Diseases and Miscellaneous Diseases* wins the reputation of "the ancestor of the medical formulary," for it records as many as 269 prescriptions, 214 kinds of medications and various forms of medicament such as decoctions, pills, powder, vinums, lotions, fumigants, eardrops, nasal drops, ointments, anal suppositories, and vaginal suppositories.

Another important medical figure in the Eastern Han dynasty, Hua Tuo (145–208 A.D.), is worth further notice. He was a famous surgeon and at the same time a master of all branches of medicine: internal medicine, surgery, gynecology, pediatrics, as well as acupuncture and moxibustion. One thousand seven hundreds years ago, he executed the earliest recorded abdominal surgery using an herbal anesthesia, *Mafei San*, which was unprecedented not only in Chinese medical history but also in the world's anesthesiological and surgical history. In his *Chinese Pharmaceutical Historical Data*, Xue Yu pointed out that Hua Tuo was the inventor of narcotics. Hua Tuo's discovery was much earlier than the British chemist Humphry Davy who discovered laughing gas (nitrous oxide) in the 18th century, earlier than American chemist G. Colton who studied the function of laughing gas on the human body in 1844, earlier than Horace Wells who conducted surgery using laughing gas in 1845, and earlier than J. Y. Simpson who relieved pains of childbirth using chloroform in 1847.

1.2.2 The Jin Dynasty (265–420 A.D.)

Chinese people have created rich diagnostic and therapeutic techniques. Among various diagnostic methods, pulsing was highly developed in the Jin dynasty (265–420 A.D.). The famous physician Wang Shuhe of the Jin dynasty composed the first monograph on sphygmology in the world, *The Pulse Classic*,[16] which elaborated the methods of pulse differentiation and classified pulse conditions into twenty-four types. Almost all types of physiological and pathological pulse conditions in today's circulatory system can be found in this book. For example, slow pulse in *The Pulse Classic* means the heart rate is fewer than sixty beats per minute, which is the pulse condition of *sinus bradycardia* in modern medicine. Such cognition has greatly influenced the development of sphygmology in the world. It was introduced to Korea and Japan in the 6th century; in the 10th century, *The Canon of Medicine* written by the Arabic physician ibn-Sīnā (980–1037) took Chinese sphygmological works as an important reference; in the 14th century, *Chinese Scientific Treasures in Ilhan* compiled by the Persian scholar Rashid al-Din al-Hamdani (1247–1318) introduced Wang Shuhe's theory of sphygmology to western countries; at the end of the 17th century, the famous British doctor John Floyer translated it into English, and thus invented the method of counting a pulse using a watch.

Among various therapeutic techniques, acumoxibustion developed rapidly early in the Jin dynasty. Huangpu Mi summarized the important contents of acumoxibustion in *Plain Questains, The Classic of Acupuncture*[17] and *Acumoxibustion on Mingtang Acupoint*[18] and compiled the earliest monograph on acumoxibustion, *The A-B Classic of Acumoxibustion*.[19] The book takes twelve meridians as the basis, determines 649 acupoints, records 880 indications of acumoxibustion, creates such techniques as directional reinforcement-reduction (a form of needle manipulation in which reinforcement or reduction is achieved by the direction of needle insertion), and discovers the taboos of acumoxibustion. The application and developmental achievements of acumoxibustion in Japan are directly relative to the introduction of *The A-B Classic of Acumoxibustion*, which is designated by the Japanese government as a required book for TCM students. In addition, it also had an impact on the acumoxibustion therapy in Korea and Europe, where the acupoints of *The A-B Classic of Acumoxibustion* were adopted.

In addition, in his medical work *A Handbook of Prescriptions for Emergencies*,[20] Ge Hong (261–341 A.D.) investigated the "itch mite," "pulmonary tuberculosis," "tuberculosis," "smallpox," "scrub typhus," and "bite by rabid dog." These are not only the earliest records in ancient Chinese medical literature, but also are the earliest in the world's lemology. The incidence and clinical features of scrub typhus, discovered by Ge Hong 1,600 years ago, was not scientifically tackled by the Japanese until the 19th century.

1.2.3 The Tang, Song, and Yuan Dynasties (618–1368 A.D.)

In the Tang, Song, and Yuan dynasties, TCM has made great achievements in diagnosis, treatment, pharmacology, medical system, and medical education.

First, *Medical Secrets of an Official*[21] written in the Tang dynasty (618–907 A.D.) shows that colorimetry, a technique of dipping the silk into urine, was used to diagnose jaundice and to judge its curative effect; one of the diagnostic standards of diabetes was "sweet urine."

Second, as to treatment, although massage therapy was originally recorded in *The Classic of Internal Medicine*, it was not until the Tang dynasty that it fully developed into an independent branch and was widely applied in internal medicine, surgery, traumatology, etc. Such a therapy was introduced to Korea and Japan not later than the Tang dynasty.

Orthopedic treatment also developed rapidly in the Tang dynasty. The manipulative restoration of the dislocated mandibular joints invented by Sun Simiao (581–682) was applied in clinical practice. *The Taoist Lin's Secret Recipes for Wounds and Bone-setting*[22] completed in the 9th century is the earliest monograph on traumatology extant in China, which shows the advanced techniques for treating fractures and dislocations. The book had much influence on resetting a broken bone by using a "ladder" device invented by Wei Yilin in the Yuan dynasty and on today's modified restoration of a dislocated shoulder. *Effective Prescriptions Handed Down for Generations*[23] written by Wei Yilin was a significant orthopedic work, in which the techniques for resetting a broken bone and fixing dislocated joints were much more advanced than those in the Tang and Song dynasties. Such techniques as fixating with four splints, fixating with bamboo hoops (for the knee), and using a curved needle to suture a wound from the inside to the outside were first recorded in Chinese orthopaedic literature. And the suspension reduction method invented by Wei Yilin is 500 years earlier than its earliest use in Europe.

Gynecology, obstetrics, and pediatrics were fully developed in the Tang and Song dynasties, and a large number of relevant monographs emerged. In 1140, *Prescriptions for Midwifery*[24] by Yu Liu recorded the invention of "the bolus for midwifery" made of rabbit brains; this mostly accords with modern science's proven method of using the posterior lobe of the pituitary to induce the contraction of the uterus. *Treatise on Infant Health and Pediatric Prescriptions*[25] discovered that neonatal tetanus and adult tetanus were the same kind of disease, and therefore invented an herbal cake with which to burn the umbilical cord to prevent neonatal tetanus. In Europe, however, it was not until 1884 that German biologist Arthur Nicolaier found that neonatal tetanus and adult tetanus were both caused by tetanus bacilli; this was some 600 years later than the relevant discovery by the Chinese in the 13th century.

Third, in the Tang and Song dynasties, TCM also made great achievements in pharmacology. The earliest pharmacopoeia issued by the Chinese government is *The Newly Revised Materia Medica* completed in 659 A.D., also known as *The Chinese Materia Medica of the Tang Dynasty*; this is some 800 years earlier than the European monumental work *Nuremberg Pharmacopoeia*. In the 7th century, mercury alloy was applied to crown teeth. It is worth mentioning that in the 11th century, the methods of preparation for urinary steroid hormones were divided into *yang* refining and *yin* refining, according to both *Well-tried Formulae by Su and Shen*[26] and *The Classified Materia Medica*.[27] Saponin precipitate steroids were successfully applied in *yang* refining in 1061 by Chinese physicians; these were first made by modern steroid chemists in the 1920s and 1930s.

Fourth, in the Tang and Song dynasties, the Chinese medical system, medical education, and medical service systems took the lead in world medicine. According to *Six Legal Documents of the Tang Dynasty*,[28] the earliest medical educational system in China was established in 443, and the professors and the assistants of imperial physicians, and other medical officers were designated by the government in the Northern Wei dynasty. In the Tang dynasty, the medical educational organization fully developed. The Office of Imperial Medical Affairs set up in the Sui dynasty was then divided into four departments: The Department of Executive, the Department of Education, the Department of Health, and the Department of Pharmaceutics. It was both an educational and a medical institute; it set courses from the basic to the advanced and organized exams every month, quarter, and year. Those who failed in the examinations would be flunked out. In the Song dynasty, the training of medical talent won much more attention and medical education was more advanced than that in the Tang dynasty. In addition, medical research was much broadened and exam regulations were much stricter. Particular importance was attached to both theoretical study and medical practice. Furthermore, medical management was much enhanced. Imperial hospitals, medical officers and other charitable organizations were established, medical education and administrative institutions were separated, and a national pharmaceutical executive was appointed.

1.2.4 The Ming and Qing Dynasties (1368–1911 A.D.)

The TCM wonder in pharmacology is *The Compendium of Materia Medica*[29], which, composed over twenty-seven years by the famous pharmacologist Li Shizhen (1518–1593) and published in 1596, recorded 1,892 kinds of medicines, 11,096 attached medical formulae and 1,160 illustrations. Its botanic classification was the most advanced in the world at that time, more than 200 years earlier than that by European botanist Carolus Linnaeus (1707–1778). It has been translated into Latin, Korean, Japanese, Russian, English, French and other languages since its publication. Charles Darwin (1809–1882) once quoted the explanation of color formation of gold fish in *The Compendium of Materia Medica* to illustrate the phenomenon of the artificial selection of animals in his work *The Origins of Mankind*. *The Compendium of Materia Medica* was called "the encyclopedia of ancient China" by Darwin thanks to its special contributions to the world's pharmacy, pharmacology, botany, and biology.

In addition, the treatment of various infectious diseases developed rapidly in the Ming and Qing dynasties. The School of Epidemic Febrile Diseases broke through Zhang Zhongjing's initiation of syndrome differentiation of infectious pestilence from the perspective of Six Meridians, and advocated syndrome differentiation according to the defensive phase, *qi* phase, nutrient phase, and blood phase, as well as the syndrome differentiation of the "*triple energizer*." These methods have been widely used in clinical practice and were the most effective methods before the discovery of antibiotics. Even nowadays, the theory of seasonal febrile disease, as well as the methods of "clearing heat to remove toxins" and "clearing nutrient phase to cool the blood," still have bright prospects for medical application.

1.3 Basic Theoretical Views of TCM

Just as Friedrich Engels pointed out in *Dialectics of Nature* that "No matter what attitudes natural scientists adopt, they are always guided by philosophy," TCM has been profoundly

1.3 Basic Theoretical Views of TCM

influenced by ancient Chinese philosophy.

1.3.1 The Outlook of Man and Nature

The TCM's outlook of man and nature is a general understanding of the relation between the human body and its natural conditions. *The Classic of Internal Medicine* states that an understanding of the natural laws enables a doctor to know more about the human body. Influenced by Chinese philosophy, TCM stresses both the unity and the correspondence between man and nature.

1.3.1.1 TCM's View about Nature

TCM's view about nature can be stated in the following four aspects, concerning its formation, inner relation, motion, and the laws of its motion.

TCM's understanding of nature begins with its recognition of *qi*, one basic philosophical notion in ancient China. It is the original substance of all things in the natural world. The ancient Chinese believed that the accumulation of *qi* forms the substance, while its dispersion results in the disappearance of substance. So *qi* and substance are unified as a whole. The *qi* theory involves the following four connotations. Firstly, the primordial *qi* can be further classified into *yin-qi* and *yang-qi* according to its nature: the light and clear *yang-qi* is hot, ascending, and active; the heavy and turbid *yin-qi* is cold, descending, and static. "Clear *yang-qi* accumulates upward to form the heaven, and turbid *yin-qi* deposits downward to form the earth" (*Plain Questions, V*). Second, the primordial *qi* can also be categorized into celestial *qi* and terrestrial *qi* in light of its location. Celestial *qi* and terrestrial *qi* interact and generate nine prefectures of the earth, four seasons of a year, 30 days in odds months, and 29 days in lunar months, and then all the things in nature. Third, the nature and quantity of *qi* determines the state of things. A case is that different diseases are caused by different pathogenic *qi* (Wu Youke, *Treatise on Pestilence*)[30]. This viewpoint confirms the materiality of nature. Accordingly, TCM, influenced by the philosophy of the ancient naive materialism, insists on the materiality of *qi* and forms the natural view of the materialistic "monism of *qi*."

The second aspect of the view of nature concerns various relations of things in nature, which can be expounded in terms of *yin-yang* and the Five Elements. The theory of *yin-yang* generalizes the relation between two relevant things, and the theory of Five Elements highlights the complicated internal structures and relations of various things. With these two theories, TCM explains the internal and external relations among various things, as well as their movement and change. It also expounds the reason why the organism can maintain the relative stabilization in its functional activities.

Third, nature is characteristic of its constant motion, propelled by the interaction of *yin-qi* and *yang-qi*. TCM holds that it is *qi* that makes the world go around, with the unceasing emergence of new things, growing from young to old, and then descending from strong to weak and finally to dead. Traditional Chinese philosophy believes that the generation and development of all things are the result of the evolution from invisible *qi* to visible substance. Influenced by this viewpoint, TCM has made a profound study on the occurrence and evolution of diseases. According to *Chiseling Open the Regularity of Qian (Heaven)*,[31] "the visible things originate from the invisible *qi*, namely, the invisible primordial *qi* is the origin of life. In the life process, the imbalanced *qi* activities inevitably cause diseases." That is, disease is also a product of the nature.

Fourth, the motion and change of nature follow such laws as spouting in spring, growing in summer, reaping in autumn, and storing in winter, which are called "the law of the universe" and "the law of changes" by *The Classic of Internal Medicine* (which will be elaborated in 5.3 The Theory of Five Elements of Chapter 5).

1.3.1.2 TCM's View about Man

First, man takes qi as essential element. For one thing, "accumulation of qi produces life while desperation of qi leads to death." The original substance of human life is called essential qi, which is produced before the birth of mankind and has the genetic characteristics. "Essential qi (congenital essence) from parents combines to produce life" (*The Classic of Internal Medicine*). According to *Spiritual Pivot*,[32] X, "human life originates from essence qi, develops into the brain and spinal cord, and finally the body is shaped. Skeletons are like the wooden pillars on the two sides of the wall, channels like the barracks connecting each other, tendons like the strings, muscles like the walls, and skins and hairs are the protector of man's bones, channels, tendons, and muscles." Human life has to depend on the nourishment and supplement of essential qi to support the endless vital activities. For another, TCM maintains that human life depends on "qi-transformation," namely the movement and change of qi as well as its relevant transformation. The ascending, descending, coming in and going out activities of qi are the basis of the life activities, so it is said that "As to animal and human beings, life will perish as long as respiration ceases; as for plant and mineral, when qi fails to ascend and descend, its vitality will wither away. Thus, where there is qi activity, there are animals' birth, growth, maturity, aging and death, as well as plants' sprouting, growth, transformation, reaping and storage" (*Plain Questions, LXVIII*).

Second, man is the unity of physique and spirit. Physique is the noumenon of life, the body. And spirit, in a broad sense, refers to the physiological and pathological manifestations of human life activities; in a narrow sense, it is the human mind and mental activities. Specifically, in TCM, the concept of spirit mainly involves the following three connotations. Spirit, in its first sense, refers to the varied functions of nature, just as Xun Zi (a representative of Confucianism at the end of the Warring States Period (475–221 B.C.)) said that the origination, growth, and change of nature are the manifestations of the vital functioning of spirit. Then it refers to all life activities of the human body. The ancient TCM holds that the human body itself is an entity of *yin-yang* opposition and unity, which promotes the motion and change of life. Last, spirit also refers to human spirit. The superior form of spiritual activity, according to the ancient Chinese, is thinking governed by the heart, the monarch of the human body. A vivid case in point is the written form of the Chinese character "想" (thinking), with "心" (heart) as its residence. The heart generates feelings by sensory contact with the outside world, and thus produces the perception and cognition of outside substances.

In addition, TCM believes that physique and spirit depend on each other, and their unity is the important guarantee of life existence. For one thing, spirit cannot exist without physique, for the material bases of spirit are qi and blood, which are also the basic components of the human body. For another, the functional activities of viscera and tissues as well as the circulation of qi and blood are governed and affected by spirit.

1.3.1.3 Correspondence between Man and Nature

It refers to the corresponding relation between the human body and nature. Such a view can be expounded from the following three aspects.

First, man is the product of nature. Namely, man originates from *qijiao*, namely the convergence of the descending celestial qi and ascending terrestrial qi.

Second, man grows on the substances that are generated by the movements and changes of celestial qi and terrestrial qi.

Third, man is directly and indirectly affected by the changes of nature. Take the physiological activity of the liver, for example. The liver regulates qi activity, stores blood, and controls the circulation of qi and blood to promote human's life function, all of which become active in spring and are synchronous with the natural changes in spring. Corresponding to nature, various viscera have their own spatial-temporal characteristics, which are generalized as "man correlates with nature, and corresponds with the shift of the sun and the moon" (*Spiritual Pivot, LXXIX*). Human physiological activities and pathological courses correspond with the obvious spatial-temporal natural condition in that, for one thing, man has the identity with all things in the universe on its material basis, which leads to the internal relation between man and nature; for another, human beings live in the place where descending celestial *qi* and ascending terrestrial *qi* converge, in which the invisible *qi* functions as inter-media to convey the changing information of the nature to the human organism.

The above view guides the medical practice of TCM and plays an important role in the understandings of physiology, pathology, diagnosis, and treatment in TCM. It promotes people to study human life, healthcare, and disease treatment against a broad natural background.

1.3.2 TCM's Physiological and Pathological Outlooks

Despite some anatomic bases, TCM's physiology and pathology are not expounded morphologically. Rather, they stress the domination of the ontology of *qi* (1.3.1.1) and the integrity of human functions, as well as the correspondence between the human body and nature.

1.3.2.1 The Physiological Outlook in TCM

One essential part of TCM physiology is *zang-xiang* theory, which concerns the physiological functions and pathological changes of various viscus and their interrelations. A man's physiological system takes five *zang*-organs as its center, coordinated by the six *fu*-organs, with *qi*, blood and the body fluid as its substantial bases. Every two *zang*-organs, *fu*-organs, as well as the *zang*-organ and *fu*-organ are closely connected by the meridians and collaterals. *Zang-fu* organs are connected with the five sense organs (eyes, tongue, mouth, nose, ear), the nine orifices (eyes, nostrils, ear canals, mouth, urethra, anus), limbs, and skeletons into an organic whole. The physiological functions of five *zang*-organs are to produce and store essence, and those of six *fu*-organs are to receive, transmit, and transform food.

Zang-xiang theory comes from the morphological cognition of the ancient anatomy. *Spiritual Pivot, XII* states that "The body of a grown-up man has skins, muscles and channels; one can inspect a living man by touching, examine a dead body by autopsy. Standards of examination are the firmness of five solid organs, the size of six hollow organs, the quantity of the cereals received, the length of the channels, and the clearness of the blood, etc."

Zang-xiang theory also comes from the long-term observation about the human physiological and pathological phenomena. For example, ancient Chinese physicians knew the close relations between the skin, nose, and lung for the observation that the symptoms of aversion to cold, nasal discharge and cough always appear, when one was invaded by cold. Besides, ancient Chinese physicians analyzed and counterproved the physiological functions of the human body from the pathological phenomena and the curative effect in the repeated medical practice. For instance, ophthalmic diseases were often cured by treating the liver, and thus people reached the physiological understanding that "the liver opens into the eyes."

The main feature of *zang-xiang* theory is holism centering around five *zang*-organs. Firstly, *zang*-organs and *fu*-organs are internally and externally related through meridians and collaterals, and thus constitute pairs of functional unit, such as the heart and small intestine, lungs and large intestine, the spleen and the stomach, the liver and the gallbladder, kidneys and the urinary bladder. Second, five *zang*-organs and their constituents, orifices and external manifestations form a whole. For example, the heart governs vessels, opens into the tongue, and manifests itself on the face; lungs govern skins, open into the nose, and manifest themselves on body hair; the spleen governs muscles, opens into the tongue and manifests itself on the lips. Thirdly, the physiological activities of five *zang*-organs are closely related to the human spirit and emotions. Human spirit, emotions, consciousness, and thinking are the functions of the human body. "The heart stores spirit, lungs store corporeal soul, the liver stores ethereal soul, the spleen stores mind and kidneys store will" (*Plain Questions, XXIII*), not because ancient Chinese physicians do not understand the function of brain, but because they integrate the human spirit and the functions of the five *zang*-organs as a whole. Fourth, the balance and coordination among five *zang*-organs, and that between *zang*-organs and constituents, orifices, spirit, and emotions are important for the human body to keep a relatively invariable and harmonious internal-external condition.

In addition to *zang-xiang* theory, meridians and collaterals as well as *qi*, blood, and body fluids are also the main contents of TCM physiology. Meridians and collaterals include *twelve regular meridians* and *eight extraordinary meridians*. They function as channels where *qi* and blood circulate to nourish organs and tissues, and as a network to connect and regulate the functions of viscera, organs, four limbs, and joints. *Qi*, blood, and body fluids, which are the basic substances to form the human body and to maintain life activities, have the functions of promoting, warming, transforming, and nourishing; they play an important role in the operation of the overall functions of the human body.

Generally, the physiological functions of *zang-fu* organs, meridians, and collaterals as well as *qi*, blood, and body fluids in TCM have surpassed their physical structures. The integrity, continuity, correlation, and mutual-transformation of these functions constitute the complexity of the human body.

1.3.2.2 TCM's Pathological Outlook

TCM holds that the opposite but unified viscera and tissues of the human body, as well as the human body and its external environment, maintain a relative dynamic *yin-yang* balance to guarantee the normal physiological activities. When the dynamic balance is damaged and cannot recover soon, diseases will occur. The causes of *yin-yang* imbalance (pathogenic factors) are *six excesses*, *seven emotions*, improper diet, overwork, pestilence, and trauma. They can be generalized into three types: "endogenous, exogenous, and other factors" (*A Handbook of Prescriptions for Emergencies*). Specifically "the endogenous ones refer to the invasion of exogenous pathogenic factors into the viscera from meridians; the exogenous ones come from the attack from skin, bringing on blood stagnation; the third is the injuries caused by sexual indulgence, cut, insect, animal bites, and the like" (*Synopsis of the Golden Chamber*).[33] This kind of classification is of much significance to differentiate diseases and provide the basis for treatment.

TCM maintains that the occurrence, development, and changes of diseases are closely related to the constitution and the functional state of the human body as well as the nature of pathogenic factors. When pathogenic factors invade the body, the struggle between vital energy and pathogenic factors will affect the relative *yin-yang* balance; the functional imbalance of *zang-fu* organs or the disorder of *qi* and blood will result in various pathological changes of the whole body or the local part. Although diseases are varied and their clinical manifestations are complex, pathogenesis mainly includes the exuberance of pathogenic factors, the declination of vital energy, the imbalance of *yin* and *yang*, the disorder of *qi* and blood, as well as the functional disorder of *zang-fu* organs, meridians, and collaterals. They are the basis for TCM to form its pathological recognition of "syndrome." As a pathological generalization of disease, "syndrome" synthesizes the complex clinical symptoms, causes, and pathogenesis. "Syndrome" includes the following contents. The first is the evidence, namely, the main clinical symptoms and pathological phenomena; the second is groups of interrelated symptoms in a certain phase of a disease; the third is the synthetic conclusion of the disease, including its etiology, pathogenesis, nature, and tendency; the fourth is the concrete pathological judgment of a disease at a certain stage in the course of its development, which also involves etiology, pathogenesis, etc. "Syndrome" is a peculiar pathological outlook in understanding the disease in TCM, and is one essential content of TSD.

1.3.3 TCM's Outlook on Health Maintenance and Treatment

The system of health maintenance and treatment gradually forms and develops based on thousands of years' clinical practice. The purpose of health maintenance is to promote health and to prevent diseases before onset and their deterioration. TCM therapeutics emphasizes such principles as "to focus on the principal cause of diseases," "to strengthen vital energy to eliminate pathogenic factors," "to regulate *yin* and *yang*," and "to select the proper therapy according to individuality, time, and geographical environment."

1.3.3.1 The Outlook of Health Maintenance in TCM

How to keep healthy, prevent diseases, and prolong life is an important content of health maintenance in TCM. The preventive idea of "treating disease before its onset" stresses taking measures in advance to prevent the occurrence or the development of diseases (*The Classic of Internal Medicine*). It can achieve twice the result with half the effort. Otherwise, treating will be as ineffective as digging wells when thirsty, or casting swords while fighting. Till now, the priority of prevention is still the basic content in China's health policy.

2,000 years ago, TCM already had the cognition of a human's life span. *Spiritual Pivot, LIV* pointed out that one hundred years should be the normal human life span. Thus, the purpose of health maintenance is "to live more than one hundred years old," and the basic method is to regulate the body and mind. For one thing, TCM believes that the state of vital energy depends on the constitution. Persons of strong constitution have the superabundance of vital energy while those of weak constitution have to suffer the insufficiency of vital energy. *Plain Questions, LXXII* said that "armed with sufficient vital energy, man can resist pathogenic factors." Therefore, the key to enhance the body against pathogenic factors is to strengthen the constitution. For another, TCM holds that emotional activities exert great influence on the physiological state and may cause pathological changes. A sudden and violent spiritual upset is often likely to lead to the disorder of *qi* activity and the imbalance between *qi* and blood, which results in disease occurrence or disease aggravation. The pleasure in one's mind can result in the harmony of *qi* activity, as well as the balance of *qi* and blood, *yin* and *yang*. *Plain Questions, I* stresses the significance of mental soundness in health maintenance: "When one is completely free from desires, ambitions and distracting thoughts, indifferent to fame and gain, he will be imbued with congenital energy; when one keeps a sound mind, how can any disease occur?"

Regular exercise is also advocated by ancient Chinese physicians to strengthen the constitution. A case in point is that Hua Tuo (145–208 A.D.), the famous physician in the Eastern Han dynasty, created a kind of gymnastics, "five fauna-mimic frolics," which are the movements in imitation of the movements of five types of wildlife – tiger, deer, bear, ape, and bird. The gymnastics shows that conforming to nature is a proper way to maintain health. Chinese doctors in later dynasties inherited this method and created more means to maintain health, such as *taiji boxing*, Eight Section Brocade (one of the most common forms of Chinese *qigong* used as exercise) and *xingyiquan* (one of the major "internal" [nèijiā] Chinese martial arts), all of which not only can strengthen one's constitution, but also have certain curative effects for many chronic diseases like chronic gastritis. Until now, they are still widely used in healthcare in China.

TCM's health maintenance also attaches importance to the regulation of daily life. "Those who keep healthy always stay in accordance with nature in daily life. They follow the principle of *yin-yang*, balance their diet, and rarely overwork." Those "who are addictive to drink, keeping idling as a life routine, or indulge in sexual pleasures, will use up their vital energy and ruin their health" (*Plain Questions, I*).

Among rich techniques of health maintenance, "conforming to nature" is especially emphasized. *Plain Questions, II* pointed out that "The law of *yin-yang* variation dominates the beginning and the end of everything as well as the birth and death of human beings. If this law is well-adapted to, man can maintain health, otherwise diseases will occur."

1.3.3.2 TCM's Therapeutic Outlook

TCM's therapeutic system gradually forms through the long-time clinical practice and the incessant summary of rich therapeutic experiences. Following are the main TCM therapeutics principles.

First, the basic principles of TCM therapeutics are "to prevent diseases before its onset" and "to prevent deterioration," namely, to keep diseases from occurring, or to stop their development and change. The reason is that "the arrival of a pathogenic wind is like a sudden storm. When it invades the human body, first skin and body hair, and then human muscles, six *fu*-organs, and finally five *zang*-organs are attacked. When five *zang*-organs are impaired, it is hard to anticipate the curative effect and the surviving rate is only 50%" (*Plain Questions, V*). That is, the early diagnosis and treatment can prevent the deterioration of disease. In *The Classic of Medical Problems*, it is further explained that "Measures must be taken to strengthen the function of the spleen in the treatment of liver disease, or to keep the spleen off pathogenic factors, for the pathological changes of the liver tend to transmit to the spleen." Such a therapeutic method is called "to treat disease before its onset," which emphasized the principle that prevention is more important than treatment.

Second, "to focus on the principal cause of disease" is also important in TCM therapeutics. The occurrence of diseases has principal and secondary causes, which can be transformed into each other with the development of diseases at their various stages, and thus it is a complicated but important task to probe into the principal cause of diseases in their dynamic changes, which is the reason why TCM advocates TSD.

Third, the key to treatment is to restore *yin-yang* balance by proper regulation, for diseases are mostly caused by the damage of the relative balance between *yin* and *yang*, whose specific manifestations are the exuberance of pathogenic factors and the declination of vital energy, as well as the discordance between the defensive phase, *qi* phase, nutrient phase, and blood phase.

Fourth, TCM stresses the overall regulating of *qi* and blood in treatment. All viscera and tissues are consubstantial in *qi* and blood, which determines that they are interdependent in physiology but mutually influential in pathology. The disease in one organ may affect or transform another. Therefore, physicians should attach importance to the regulation of *qi* and blood. For example, the deficiency of *qi* and blood can cause dysmenorrhea, anorexia, and abdominal pain, which can be treated by supplementing *qi* and blood.

Finally, TCM holds that proper therapies are also decided according to individuality, especially some genetic constitutions, as well as seasonal and geographical environment, which may affect the occurrence, development and prognosis of a disease. Such a view is the manifestation of the medical holism. For example, muscular interstices are believed loose in spring and autumn, when it turns warmer and *yang-qi* gradually elevates. Therefore, to avoid excessive purgation and the damage to *yin-qi*, herbs acrid in taste and warm in nature cannot be used in a large dosage even for wind-cold attack. In autumn and winter, the muscular interstices are dense because it becomes colder, *yin* becomes predominant, and *yang* turns deficient, and thus in these two seasons cold-natured herbs should be used cautiously except for serious heat syndrome.

Only when doctors completely grasp TCM's therapeutic principles, can clinical practice be more reasonable and thus more effective.

CHAPTER 2
Theoretical System of TCM: Formation and Characters

Objectives & Requirements
1. Social-cultural background of the establishment of TCM's theoretical system.
2. Ancient philosophy influencing the formation of TCM's theoretical system.
3. TCM's disciplinary properties as a natural science and a humanistic-social science.
4. TCM's unique academic characters different from other natural sciences.

Key Concepts
It took a long time for the theoretical system of TCM to come into being. The Spring and Autumn Period (722–481 B.C.) and the Warring States Period (475–221 B.C.) are a time of great social changes, and are imbued with various schools of thought, which provides a favorable social and cultural condition for the development of medicine. Meanwhile, the explorations into the man-nature relation and the mystery of the human body gradually promotes medicine to evolve from experiential accumulation to theoretical reflection, and then to the formation of a theoretical system. Based on the thoughts of pre-Qin scholars, and the ancient philosophical theories like *yin-yang* and the Five Elements, TCM formed its own physiological and pathological cognitions like *zang-xiang*, *qi*, blood, and meridians and collaterals.

Originated from the ancient society and closely related to the local geography and traditional academic thoughts, TCM not only has its own multidisciplinary properties like other natural sciences, humanistic-social sciences, and philosophies, but also has the same concern of modern medicine for their same research objective, the human body.

2.1 The Formation of the Theoretical System of TCM

The establishment of the initial theoretical system of TCM benefits from ancient China's vigorous social culture, philosophy, and medical practice.

2.1.1 The Promotion of Social Culture

The Warring States Period (475–221 B.C.) is one historical period when China experienced great social transformations, that is, slavery society was overthrown by feudal society, and accordingly the slavery owner class was replaced by the newly risen landlord class. The change of production relations and the improvement of production techniques enormously promoted productivity, which brought about the rapid development of the agriculture-relevant scientific techniques, astronomy, calendar system, and agronomy. Meanwhile, a philosophical state of "a hundred flowers blossoming and a hundred schools of thought contending" appeared, which produced varied academic schools, such as Confucianism, Taoism, Mohism, Legalism, Logicians, and the *Yin-yang* School. Among them, Confucian, Taoist, and the *Yin-yang* School had the greatest effect on the formation and development of TCM. Confucian morality had a great influence on the ancient medical ethic; Taoist exploration into life, understanding of the essence, *qi*, and spirit, as well as the theory of health maintenance had a significant effect on TCM's view of life; the theories of *Yin-yang* and Five Elements shed great light on human's physiology and pathology. In addition, atheist Xun Kuang (313–238 B.C.) put forward the thought of "conquering the nature under the guidelines of the objective laws," which exerted a positive influence on TCM in its struggling with witchcraft in the pre-Qin Period, and impelled the development of TCM in the right direction.

In the Eastern Han dynasty (25–220 A.D.), the outstanding thinker Wang Chong (27–97 A.D.) criticized such idealist fallacies as predestination and ghosts, insisting that *qi* be the essential source of all things in the universe. He further put forward atheism and correctly expounded the body-spirit relationship, all of which laid a materialistic foundation for TCM.

2.1.2 Experiential Accumulation

Since primitive society, the medical practitioners and researchers in China had accumulated rich medical experiences, which laid a foundation for the establishment of TCM's theoretical system.

Early in the Western Zhou dynasty (1046–771 B.C.), the names of some diseases were first determined. For example, thirty-eight types of diseases were recorded in *The Classics of Mountains and Rivers*, and twenty-three of them had their fixed names.

By the Spring and Autumn Period (722–481 B.C.), wine, decoction and even the poisonous medicine had been applied or invented to treat diseases. Meanwhile, the therapeutic techniques such as acupuncture and moxibustion had been widespread. Besides, both the initial formation of the theories of *yin-yang* and the Five Elements and the appearance of the specialized physicians provide a favorable condition for the establishment of TCM's theoretical system. For example, the theory of etiology and pathogenesis sprouted at that time. That *Zuo Commentary*[34] accounted for "six kinds of *qi*" is a good case. Six kinds of *qi*, i.e., cold, heat, wind, rain, gloominess, and drought, are six exogenous factors, the excess of which may respectively lead to cold diseases, heat diseases, head diseases, gastrointestinal diseases, depression, and irritability.

In the Warring States Period (475–221 B.C.), diagnostic methods came into being, thanks to the efforts of specialized physicians and large quantity of experiential accumulation. The Four Diagnostic Methods, i.e., inspection, auscultation and olfaction, interrogation and pulse taking, and palpation were commonly applied at that time. Besides, varied therapeutic methods like acupuncture, moxibustion, and massage were fully developed. What's more, psychotherapy was also invented to treat diseases by changing the patients' mood. A record in *Lv's Spring and Autumn Annals*[35] goes as follows. Wen Zhe, a famous physician in the Warring States Period, managed to cure a Qi Ming marquis of hypochondria with the method of provocation to promote the blood circulation. In addition, *A Collection of 52 Prescriptions*,[36] a silk medical book excavated from Mawangdui[37] recorded 103 names of diseases (concerning internal medicine, surgery, gynecology, pediatrics, ophthalmology, and otorhinolaryngology, and so on), 247 types of medicines and 283 kinds of prescriptions.

In the Qin and Han dynasties (221 B.C.–220 A.D.), based on the accumulation of medical experiences, TCM's theoretical system was primarily established, with *The Classic of Internal Medicine* as a symbol.

2.1.3 The Observation of Life Phenomena

Based on the observation of life phenomena, TCM forms the concept of holism, under the guidance of which, the theory of *zang-xiang* and the theory of meridians and collaterals are gradually formed.

TCM's holism, which covers the integrity of the human body itself and the unity of man and nature, is formed through the long-term observations of human physiological and pathological phenomena as well as the influence of the natural conditions on the human body.

2.1 The Formation of the Theoretical System of TCM

For one thing, without today's advanced apparatus, ancient physicians detected the physiological functions and pathological changes of internal organs through their outer manifestations. They realized that certain symptoms were caused by the malfunction of a certain inner organ, and therefore could be relieved by regulating the physiological function. For instance, the symptoms of asthma, nasal discharge, and a distension sensation in the chest indicate the malfunction of respiration dominated by the lungs, and thus certain acupoints such as Shaoshang LU 11 and Yuji LU 10 or pungent-spicy herbs like *Herba Ephedrae* that are used to regulate the function of lungs are effective in relieving the above symptoms. In this way, *zang-xiang* theory was gradually formed.

For another, the ancient Chinese also recognized the relation between man and nature by observing the influence of seasons and climates on human physiological activities and pathological changes. It is observed by *Zhou Li* that "headache often occurs in spring, scabies in summer, malaria in autumn, and cough in winter."

Guided by the concept of holism, the theory of meridians and collaterals was also gradually formed. By observing patients' reaction to acupuncture, ancient physicians discovered the transmitting route of needle sense, which is the objective foundation of the theory of meridians and collaterals. Under the guidance of holism, it was believed that some connected channels were bound to exist among *zang-fu* organs, and between *zang-fu* organs and superficial tissues. In practice, the following meridians and collaterals system were discovered: Twelve meridians, Eight extra meridians, Branches of twelve meridians, Tendons of twelve meridians, and Twelve cutaneous regions. Thus the theory of meridians, and collaterals was preliminarily established, which furthers the understanding of the integrity of the human body.

2.1.4 The Penetration of Philosophical Ideas

In the unprecedented invigorated academic atmosphere of the pre-Qin Period, the naive materialism and dialectics were developed, which had a positive influence on the development of the theoretical system of TCM. Among various theories, essence-*qi*-spirit theory, *yin-yang* theory, and Five Elements theory are essential to TCM.

2.1.4.1 Essence-*Qi*-Spirit Theory

The theory of essence, *qi* and spirit, which belongs to the naive materialism, influences the establishment of a materialistic life view in TCM positively.

In the Warring States Period, philosophers believed that all visible things in the universe originated from the invisible *qi*. In the Eastern Han dynasty, materialists regarded *qi* as the most primal substance, and everything including a human being was formed from *qi*. As what Wang Chong indicated in *On Balance*,[38] "the condensation of *qi* forms human beings."

Essence, according to TCM, is the essential substance constituting the human body and maintaining life activities. In a broad sense, it generally refers to *qi*, blood, body fluid, and essential substances from foodstuff. Just as *Spiritual Pivot, X* says, "The essence is formed first, and then it develops into brain and spinal cord, and finally the human body." Without essence there will be no life.

As to spirit, the ancient materialists believed that it was an internal and dynamic power for the development and changes of everything. Human spirit is manifested in the form of consciousness and thinking. It will disappear when one dies.

These three elements are interrelated. First, spirit is generated from essence. "When *qi* and blood are harmonious, one's nutrient *qi* and defensive *qi* are unimpeded, with his five *zang*-organs being shaped and spirit being stored in the heart[31] endowing him with thought and will" (*Spiritual Pivot, LIV*). Second, the combination of spirit and body is an important premise of the life existence. The body is often compared to a house, where the spirit is the dominator.

2.1.4.2 The Theory of *Yin-yang*

The doctrine of *yin-yang* in the ancient philosophy also falls into the ancient materialism and dialectics. The primary connotations of *yin* and *yang* only refer to the location of objects relevant to the sun. Facing the sun is called *yang*, otherwise it is *yin*. Then all natural phenomena in the universe can be termed as *yin* or *yang*. So is the most primal substance, *qi*. In the Spring and Autumn Period and the Warring States Period, ancient Chinese believed that all natural phenomena were the result of interactions between *yin* and *yang*, even the fall of aerolite and the occurrence of earthquakes. "The interaction of *yin* and *yang* generates everything in the universe" (*Yi Zhuan*:[40] *Xi Ci*), "the combination of the *yin-qi* and *yang-qi* generates everything and their interconnection produces changes" (*Hsun Tzu*:[41] *on Rites*). Gradually, a unique *yin-yang* theory in TCM was formed by combining the doctrine of *yin-yang* in the ancient philosophy with medical practices. For one thing, it is used to explain human physiological functions and pathological changes. For example, "*yin-yang* balance ensures the normal physiological state," and "the *yin-yang* imbalance causes pathological changes." For another, it also guides the clinical diagnosis and treatment. For instance, "distinguishing *yin* from *yang* is the key to diagnose," and "the therapeutic method of regulating *yin* and *yang* is effective in clinical practice." The theory of *yin-yang* penetrated every corner of medicine from theory to clinic, and thus has become an important part in the theoretical system of TCM.

2.1.4.3 The Theory of Five Elements

The theory of Five Elements is a natural philosophy in ancient China, which influences traditional Chinese medicine deeply and widely. Five Elements in ancient China refer to such indispensable substances as wood, fire, earth, metal, and water. That is why Five Elements were originally called "five materials." Gradually, Five Elements are used to summarize the properties of things: water is of the property of moistening and flowing downward; fire is of the nature of flaming upward; wood is characterized of being flexed and extended; metal is characteristic of changing and reforming; and earth is where crops grow. Five Elements restrain and promote each other. The order of interrestraint among Five Elements (interrestraint means that one thing can inhibit the generation and function of another) was first affirmed by Zou Yan (324–250 B.C.) in the Warring States Period, and the order of interpromotion among Five Elements (interpromotion means that one thing bears the effect of promoting or generating another thing) was basically formed in *Guan Zi*[42] and *Lv's Spring and Autumn Annals*. The theory of Five Elements, which is applied in TCM, is mainly used to expound human physiology, pathology, diagnosis, and treatment. In addition, for the concept of holism, the integrity of the human body itself as well as the unity of man and nature can be elucidated in terms of Five Elements and such laws as interpromotion and interrestraint (which will be elaborated in Chapter 4).

To sum up, based on the accumulation of rich clinical experiences and guided by the theories of essence-*qi*-spirit, *yin-yang*, and Five Elements, ancient physicians established the theoretical system of TCM. Therefore, its formation has distinctive features of the times, which symbolizes the development of TCM from scattered experiences to systematic theories.

2.2 The Disciplinary Properties of TCM

TCM, one of the most important traditional schools of world medicine, is often mentioned in the same breath with modern medicine. Its special medical theories and disciplinary properties have a great effect on modern science.

2.2 The Disciplinary Properties of TCM

2.2.1 Multidisciplinary Properties: Natural Science, Humanistic-Social Science, and Philosophy

2.2.1.1 TCM's Property of Natural Science

TCM's property of natural science can be expounded in terms of its material nature and its relation with other branches of natural science.

TCM is the science that focuses on the essence of life and the laws of human life's change, namely, laws of human physiology, pathology, medical maintenance, and disease treatment. All of these are determined by the physical constituents of life such as *qi*, *yin*, *yang*, and Five Elements, though they may be invisible. First, TCM regards *qi* as the origin of life. It believes that the universe including human beings is of material property, for it is formed by *qi*. For one thing, the normality of *qi* keeps the human body in a healthy state, while its abnormality in quantity or motion results in pathological changes. For example, the gradual insufficiency of *qi* causes depletion, and its dispersion or exhaustion leads to death. For another, pathogenic factors (evil *qi*) are of material property also. For instance, *six excesses* (wind, cold, summer-heat, dampness, dryness, and heat) that cause exogenous diseases are imperceptible but material. The etiology of TCM mainly discusses the characteristics and laws of these pathogenic factors, their clinical manifestations, and the measures of prevention.

Second, TCM regards *yin-yang* and Five Elements as the theoretical bases of *zang-xiang*, meridians, collaterals, and syndromes. Specifically, the human body is an entity composed of the opposite *yin* and *yang* of various levels; if the relative equilibrium between *yin* and *yang* is damaged, man will be sick; if *yin* and *yang* separate, man will die. TCM also forms the physiological and pathological systems centering around five *zang*-organs, by combining five *zang*-organs (pertaining to Five Elements) respectively with the related five constituents (tendons, vessels, muscles, skin, and bones), five sense organs (eyes, tongue, mouth, nose, and ears) and five emotions (anger, joy, contemplation, grief, and fear). It manifests the holism of the human body.

Additionally, the natural property of TCM is also shown in its close connection with other branches of natural science. The natural world provides essential conditions for human beings to grow, but on the other hand it also affects human physiological functions directly or indirectly. The achievements of other natural sciences, such as geography, phonology, agronomy, biology, botany, mineralogy, military study, mathematics, and metallurgy have all shed some light on human life phenomena and therefore could be borrowed to further medical study. For example, meteorology has promoted the establishment of the theory of *six excesses*; with the aid of geographic knowledge, ancient physicians proposed the detailed therapeutic principles based on the local conditions; even rich mathematical knowledge was also mentioned in *The Classic of Internal Medicine*: The number of "five" is essential to the formation of the universe and human beings are no exception. Like other things, they are composed of five kinds of substance (wood, fire, earth, metal, and water), and the human body is composed of five *zang*-organs, five constituents, five sense organs, and so on.

2.2.1.2 TCM's Property of Humanistic-social Science

TCM's property of natural science is easily understood for its biological mechanism in the aspects of physiology, pathology, diagnosis, and treatment. However, its social attributes are likely to be ignored, which may cause errors in diagnosis and treatment sometimes.

First, society may bring about many medical problems to human beings. It is observed that the physiological functions of the human body vary with the social and cultural background. *Spiritual Pivot, V* states that "princes and nobles eat meat every day, and therefore their bodies are feeble, and their blood circulation is rapid and slippery." That is to say, the privileged social status of the ruling class and the dissolute and depraved life may lead to their special constitution. And therefore, just as the famous physician Li Zhongzi (1588–1655) in the Ming dynasty advocated, "The rich and the poor ought to be medically treated differently," which endows TCM with some features of social science.

Second, TCM also tries to reveal the social root of many diseases. Some diseases result from the turbulence of society, political corruption, famine, war, economic depression, or harmful customs. *Hou Han Shu* recorded a serious epidemic disease in 161 A.D. The duke Liu Tao commented that it was heavy tax and labor as well as lack of diet and rest that led to the disaster.

Third, TCM also concerns the influence of interpersonal relationships and an individuals' social role on one's health. The famous physician Zhu Zhenheng (1281–1358) has ever pointed out in *Ge Zhi Yu Lun*[43] that mammary cancer is very likely to occur among women who are depressed out of prolonged inharmonious family relationships. *Plain Questions, LXXVII* also points out that a sudden declining of an individual's social and financial status may cause severe physical and mental diseases. All these cognitions show that TCM has already penetrated into the social domain.

2.2.1.3 TCM's Philosophical Property

Any science, as history proves, cannot develop without the guidance of philosophy. Its epistemology determines the research methodology, developing direction and relevant theories. It is the same case for TCM, which is closely related to ancient Chinese philosophies.

Ancient Chinese philosophy not only provides epistemological instruction, but also becomes the concrete academic contents of TCM. Taoist doctrines like primordial *qi*, *yin-yang*, and Five Elements all attempt to promulgate the essence of the world. Guided by these doctrines, TCM developed its concept of holism (in Chapter 4), namely, for one thing, the human body is an integrated whole and one part will affect and be affected by others; for another, man and the outside world are unified in that as one part of the world, human beings have to adapt themselves to nature. In terms of holism, TCM created its special techniques in physiology, pathology, diagnosis, and treatment, like treating external diseases with internal therapy, regulating *yin* and *yang*, and TSD. *The Classic of Internal Medicine* elaborates the physiological phenomenon and the pathological process of the human body with the philosophical notion of *yin-yang*, which is used to explain the attributes and interrelation of the correlated physiological constituents or two aspects of one constituent, and created some unique terminologies in TCM like "balance between *yin* and *yang*," "interdependence between *yin* and *yang*," and "hyperactivity of *yang* due to asthenia of *yin*."

In summary, TCM is a comprehensive production of medical practice itself and has received enlightenments from other varied sciences, and therefore has multidisciplinary properties.

2.2.2 TCM: Both Basic and Applied Disciplines

TCM is of the characters of basic discipline in that it is a systematic study on the fundamental laws of life itself. Based on the accumulation of a large amount of medical experiences and rational reflections on human physiology, pathology, diagnosis, and treatment, TCM has acquired a unique cognition on the general law of life formation and development, the relations between life activities and their external environment, the structures of the human body and their interrelationships, the physiological activities and pathological manifestations of various organs, various pathogenic factors and their respective characteristics, as well as the pathogenesis and relevant therapeutic principles.

Life, according to *The Classic of Internal Medicine*, originates from the combination of parental essence, grows by unceasingly absorbing nutrients from the placenta, turns mature

2.2 The Disciplinary Properties of TCM

by inhaling fresh air through lungs, and transforms foods into nutrients for metabolism through the spleen and stomach. The abnormality of any of these processes may endanger human health and even cause death. The general laws of human growth are elaborated in *The Classic of Internal Medicine*. Females experience several growing stages with about seven years as a unit. At the age of seven, permanent teeth appear to replace deciduous ones and hair grows in a rapid speed; at the age of 14, with the arrival of menarche, female teenagers begin to have the physiological ability to reproduce; at the age of 21, growth slows down or even stops; at the age of 28, physiological functions are at their climax; at the age of 35, physiological functions start declining; at the age of 42, women begin to age with haggard faces and white hair appearing; and at the age of 49, reproductive function begins to fail with the reach of menopause. Males experience several growing stages with eight years as a unit. They begin to replace deciduous teeth with permanent teeth at the age of 8, have the ability to reproduce with the coming of occasional spermatorrhea at 16, stop growing at the age of 24, have the most powerful physiological functions at the age of 32, experience physiological decline at 40, start to age at 56, and enter the senescence phase at the age of 64.

The above understandings not only reflect the basic laws of human birth, growth, maturity, aging, and death, but also lay down the important criterions for an organism's physical conditions, like hair growing and the reproductive function, which is still of highly scientific value until now. Based on these understandings, TCM explores the intrinsic mechanism of human growth and aging, and discovers that the life process is closely related to the "*tiangui*" (*Plain Questions*). Such understandings shed great light on scientific research and clinical practice.

In addition to the exploration of life growth, TCM also investigates the pathogenesis. *The Classic of Internal Medicine* reveals that disease results from the conflicts of the two aspects of a contradiction. Under normal circumstances, human beings have "healthy qi" to protect themselves from pathogenic factors. However, the human body may be affected by various pathogenic factors, i.e. "evil qi." Disease occurs when healthy qi fails to defeat evil qi. The struggle runs through the whole process of disease occurring and progressing. This understanding macroscopically reveals the essence of diseases.

All the above show that TCM has paid attention to the study of the basic medical problems, and has established its unique theoretic system. These all make TCM of the characteristics of basic discipline.

TCM's features of applied discipline are shown in its applications in clinic, preventive medicine, pharmacology, diet therapy, and forensic medicine.

TCM's clinical achievements are extremely prominent. As early as the Spring and Autumn Period, Bian Que (407–310 B.C.), a famous physician, managed to apply various effective techniques like stone needle, acupuncture, moxibustion, massage, medicine and surgery to cure various diseases in internal medicine, surgery, pediatrics, gynecology, ophthalmology, and otorhinolaryngology. In the 2nd century, Hua Tuo executed abdominal surgery using an herbal anesthesia, *Mafei San*, and was well-known for curing Cao Cao (the prime minister of Wei Leud State in the Han dynasty) of head wind-syndrome with acupuncture. Almost at the same time, Zhang Zhongjing came up with the theory of the six meridians to differentiate exogenous febrile diseases and the theory of *zang-fu* organs to distinguish miscellaneous diseases, which are widely used nowadays. Later, ancient physicians treated scabies and malignant ulcers with mercurial, and advocated nutritional therapy, e.g., using soybean and milk to treat beriberi; using animals' liver to cure night blindness; using *Sargassum* to treat goiter; and applying brains of dogs suffering from rabies to wounds to prevent rabies in the 3rd century. All of these clinical practices have been proved reasonable and scientific by modern science.

TCM also makes a great success in preventive medicine. Early in the Zhou dynasty (1046–256 B.C.), hygienic systems were set up. In the Qin dynasty (221–206 B.C.), pesthouses for lepra came into being. In the Han dynasty (206 B.C.–220 A.D.), both "Daoyin exercise" and "Five fauna-mimic frolics" were popular in physical training. The study of epidemic diseases reached a certain degree in the Eastern Jin dynasty (317–420 A.D.), when the earliest account of the cause, distribution, infection, and prevention of smallpox, cholera, and tsutsugamushi, etc., appeared. A case is that the living form, clinical characters, way of infection, prognosis, and measures of prevention of tsutsugamushi were precisely described by Ge Hong (1152–1237), 1,600 years earlier than that in Western medicine. In the Song dynasty (960–1279 A.D.), the technique of man-pox vaccination was proved effective in controlling the rage of smallpox, which contributed a great deal to the modern immunology.

In the field of pharmacology, the earliest national pharmacopoeia in the world was finished in the early years of the Tang dynasty (618–907 A.D.), 840 years earlier than Europe. And the most influential pharmacy monograph is *The Compendium of Materia Medica*, written by Li Shizhen (1518–1593) in the Ming dynasty (1368–1644 A.D.). Since then, it has been translated into many languages, and there are more than ten English editions.

As for diet therapy, *Principles of Correct Diet*[44] appeared in the Yuan dynasty (581–1368 A.D.), elaborated various food taboos for pregnant women and daily healthcare, introduced the cooking techniques of high-nutrition foods, and also discussed nutrition therapy, food safety, and food poisoning. For its scientific values, the book was highly regarded by the famous British science and technology history scholar, Dr. Joseph Needham.

The forensic medicine in TCM is also outstanding. Early in the 10th century, the earliest books on forensic medicine appeared and by the Song dynasty (960–1279 A.D.), such books had been published in large volume. For example, *Xi Yuan Lu*,[45] written by Song Ci (1186–1249), was considered the first systematic forensic medical monograph in the world, which elaborated the dissection of the human body, autopsy, scene investigation, the cause of death appraisal, the analysis of poison used in suicide or murder, and the techniques in first aid and disintoxication. This book has been translated into Korean, Japanese, English, German, French, Dutch, and other languages, and has exerted great influence on the world of forensic medicine.

TCM is the product of medical practice and theoretical reflection, and therefore is characteristic of both basic discipline and applied discipline. These two characters are inseparable and mutual-promoting.

For one thing, basic theoretical study of medical problems is based on clinical observation and practice. Theoretical reflections are promoted by specific problems in practice. For example, through the long-term observation, ancient physicians realized that people in different regions differ in physiological functions and pathological changes because of the different geographical location, weather condition and living habit, and thus arrived at the theory of "treatment in accordance with local conditions," namely, as for the same disease, patients in different regions should be treated differently. Besides, only in practice can theoretical reflections be proved and verified. TCM adopts the concept of holism to observe life phenomena. It is a macroscopic perspective, stressing the inner and external connection between different things; it is also a dynamic perspective, observing its object as a changing one. Such cognitions of life cannot be obtained suddenly; they have experienced hundreds or even thousands of years of reflection and practical verification to make up the gap between theory and application.

For another, medical practice should be guided by medical theories, especially its updating achievements. For instance, without the guidance of the theory of meridians and collaterals as well as the theory of "meridian tropism of drugs," the remarkable curative effect in acupuncture cannot be achieved. The theory of meridians and collaterals holds that since the meridians run along certain routes and pertain to certain viscera, there is a special relationship between different parts of a body and their internal organs. Take the headache for example. It may appear in different parts of the head, connected with different meridians: pain in the forehead is related to the *Yangming* meridian; pain in both sides of the head is related to the *Shaoyang* meridian; and pain in the nape is often related to the *Taiyang* meridian. Such a fact lays the foundation for the correct and effective treatment. The theory of "meridian tropism of drugs" believes that each drug can enter one or more meridians, so based on syndrome differentiation, clinically drugs can be selected according to their state of "meridian tropism" to treat diseases so as to improve the curative effect. Again take headache for example. A headache concerning the *Taiyang* meridian should be treated with *Rhizoma et Radix Notopterygii*; that in relation to the *Yangming* meridian should be treated with *Radix Angelicae Dahuricae*; and that concerning the *Shaoyang* meridian with *Radix Bupleuri*, because these drugs enter these meridians respectively. Only under theoretical guidance, can the safety and effect of these medical applications be guaranteed.

As for the relationship between basic research and application, for one thing, the advancement of TCM in application depends on the new achievements in basic research. For another, the problems encountered in clinical application are the objects of study and impetus in basic research, promoting the theoretical development of TCM.

CHAPTER 3

Clinical System of TCM: Formation and Development

Objectives & Requirements
1. Motives of TCM's development.
2. Earlier epistemology and therapeutic views of diseases.
3. Law of disease.
4. Law of symptom.
5. Law of prescription-and-syndrome-based medication.
6. Clinical practice of Treatment Based on Syndrome Differentiation (TSD).
7. Relationship between TCM's theoretical system and clinical system.

Key Concepts
Through the long-term accumulation of practical experiences and mutual promotion of theory and practice, TCM has developed into a relatively complete academic system. Its unique clinical system consists of four parts: medical theory, principle, prescription, and herb. A comprehensive understanding of its academic noumenon, TSD, its history and content, can further our cognition about TCM's clinical system.

"Medical activities," just as Ivan Petrovich Pavlov pointed out, "began with the birth of human beings." That is, man's cognition of the occurrence, development and treatment of diseases starts very early in human society. Such ancient medical fables as "Fuxi[46] tasted hundreds of herbs and made *jiuzhen* to rescue people from dying" (*Age of Empires*)[47] and "traditional Chinese medicine appeared after Shennong tasted various herbs" (*Shi Ji Gang Jian*)[48] show that medical knowledge in the ancient times originates from people's productive activities and living practice. This chapter will turn to famous Chinese medical works to investigate how ancient Chinese come to learn disease and how TCM's clinical system is formed.

3.1 Accumulation of Clinical Experiences

3.1.1 Primitive Cognition of Disease

The oracle bone script[49] found in Yinxu[50] bears the earliest record about how the ancient Chinese learn about disease. The script shows that ancient people's understanding of disease begins with their intuitionist cognition of single posture or superficial symptoms. A case is that the symbol "爿" (疒), interpreted by Yang Shuda[51] as "病"(illness), is the icon of a person lying on the bed, and records with "疒" as one part have something to do with the symptoms of diseases. First, there are many hieroglyphs that depict the tumefaction of the breast, collare swelling, dizziness, nightmare, and so on. Second, there are some descriptions of the disease location such as "疒首" (cephalic diseases), "疒目" (ophthalmic diseases), "疒耳" (aural diseases), "疒自" (nasal diseases), "疒止" (foot diseases), and "疒腹" (abdominal diseases), for the Chinese characters "首", "目", "耳", "自", "止", and "腹" means head, eye, ear, nose, foot, and abdomen respectively. Third, there are many diseases recorded according to their main characteristics, such as "malaria," "scabies," "parasitic infestation," and "caries." Ancient Chinese also gained some therapeutic experiences like pressing a tender spot with hands or puncturing the location of the illness with sharp tools to relieve pains.

However, people in the Shang dynasty (1600–1046 B.C.) believe in god and owe the causes of all diseases to ghosts. That is why the therapeutic experiences are always mixed with prayer and sacrifice.

3.1.2 From Witches' Practice to Medical Treatment

Since the Western Zhou dynasty (1046–771 B.C.), Chinese medicine, in spite of the dominant influence of witch doctors, the extensive accumulation of clinical practical experiences, especially the knowledge of medicinal herbs, has gradually changed people's primitive understanding about diseases. Even the Chinese literature classic, *The Book of Songs*, recorded more than one hundred kinds of Chinese medicinal herbs.

The further medical progress was shown in *The Classic of Mountains and Rivers*. First, disease terminology based on characteristics appeared. Among thirty-eight diseases recorded, twenty-three have their fixed names (such as abdominal mass, goiter, hemorrhoids, scabies, carbuncle, malaria, and pestilence): twelve are named according to their symptoms (such as abdominal pain, vomiting, and deafness); three are of relatively general names (the liver diseases, abdominal diseases, as well as pectoral and abdominal diseases). Second, curable effects of 120 kinds of medicines have been described in many chapters of *The Classic of Mountains and Rivers*. For example, "human beings can be protected from poison by eating auris mouse (a kind of beast like mouse)," "people can prevent the pectoral and abdominal diseases by taking the elephant's skeleton poisoned by cobra venom" and "Feiyi (a kind of bird) can be used to treat pestilence." Third, people's cognition of medicine has improved a lot, either. They found that one disease can be treated with several medicines, and one medicine can treat many diseases. For instance, there are seven kinds of medicines for ophthalmic diseases and four kinds of medicines for hemorrhoids.

In conclusion, from the primitive understanding of diseases in the oracle bone script to the extensive accumulation of medical knowledge in the Western Zhou dynasty, people had been able to describe the symptoms, name special diseases and record some medicines, which meant that the medical practice had gradually changed from witches' practice to medical treatment. However, in this period, medical practice was still the accumulation of simple experiences, which was characteristic of the understanding of a single symptom of a disease and a single function of a medicine.

3.1.3 Medication Development: From Single-Symptom-and-Single-Medicine-Based Medication to Compound-Symptom-and-Prescription-Based Medication

The medical book unearthed from Mawangdui is a symbol for Chinese medication to develop from single-symptom-and-single-medicine-based practice to compound-symptom-and-prescription-based one.

First, symptoms were not single but compound. For example, disease of the spleen meridian of the foot *taiyin* is manifested as the halluces' disablement, femoral pain, abdominal pain, abdominal distention and anorexia. Secondly, in terms of etiology, a disease can be attributed to the natural factors such as *qi*, wind, and dampness. Third, as to treatment, according to the medication experiences recorded in *A Collection of 52 Prescriptions*, physicians in the Han dynasty mostly treat a disease with a prescription composed of various medicines. In addition, pharmacotherapy has broadened to cover decoction, external application, fumigating with herbs, and demibain; the therapeutic method has been enriched to include moxibustion, massage, and operation.

Although the relations among compound symptoms are not illustrated well and the use of prescriptions and medicines recorded shows no regularity, the comprehensive cognition of complex symptoms and the application of prescriptions go beyond the original level of experience. First, the use of prescriptions was popular in the Han dynasty (*Wuwei Wooden Fragments with the Han Dynasty's Medical Inscription*).[52] For example, "the prescription to treat exogenous febrile disease" and "the prescription to relieve dysuria" were widely applied in clinical practice. Second, the use of prescriptions and medicines was gradually standardized, for instance, *Zhi Bai Bing Fang*[53] records that the prescription to treat *fuliang* is composed of *Radix et Rhizoma Rhei*, *Radix Scutellariae*, *Radix Paeoniae Rubra*, niter, *Cortex Cinnamomi*, beak, *Halloysitum Rubrum*, *Haematitum*, *Semen Phaseoli*, and *Excrementum Bombycis*. Such an example shows that TCM's medication has developed from a single medicine based on a single symptom to the prescription based on compound symptoms. These experiences set the practical basement for TSD.

3.2 Exploration of Disease's Cause and Law

The development of medical treatment, from prayer and sacrifice to medication of a single medicine based on a single symptom, then to medication of the prescription based on compound symptoms, and finally to treatment based on symptom differentiation, all prove that it is continuous medical practice and constant experience accumulation that promote TCM's clinical progress.

3.2.1 *The Classic of Internal Medicine* and *The Classic of Medical Problems*: Explorations of the Cause and Law of Disease

The Classic of Internal Medicine tries to explore the causes of diseases and advocates syndrome differentiation in treatment.

For one thing, *The Classic of Internal Medicine* attributes diseases to exogenous factors, emotional reasons, the disorders of meridians and viscera, and abnormal pathological changes of *yin-yang*, *qi*, blood, and body fluid. For example, we can find the etiology and pathogenesis records in *The Classic of Internal Medicine*: "Various diseases result from such exogenous pathogenic factors as dryness, dampness, cold, summer-heat, wind and heat, excessive emotions, immoderate diet and abnormal daily life"; "when food and drink of improper temperature are taken in, it may cause diseases in stomach and intestine, so food can hurt six *fu*-organs"; "pathogenic dampness retaining in the body will damage skin, muscle and meridians."

For another, syndromes of a kind of disease are differentiated by the causes in *The Classic of Internal Medicine*. For example, febrile disease can be categorized into exogenous febrile disease and endogenous febrile disease. And even the syndromes of an exogenous febrile disease may be different. "When pathogenic wind, cold and dampness attack the human body at the same time, they will cause obstruction syndrome (rheumatism): the predominant pathogenic wind will result in migratory obstructive syndrome; the exuberant pathogenic cold will bring on painful obstructive syndrome; and the predominant pathogenic dampness will lead to damp obstructive syndrome" (*Plain Questions*, Chapter 43).

Therefore, *The Classic of Internal Medicine* holds that the physician should decide the therapeutic principles and select the proper therapy based on syndrome differentiation, for example, "treating cold syndrome with warm therapy and heat syndrome with cold therapy" (*Plain Questions*, Chapter 74).

Like *The Classic of Internal Medicine*, *The Classic of Medical Problems* also tries to elucidate the reasons for diseases. For example, "precordial pain can be caused by either the deficiency of blood in the heart, or the stagnation of *qi* and blood." However, unlike *The Classic of Internal Medicine*, it also expounds specific etiology and pathogenesis in the terms of "three excess and three aexcess," "five kinds of pathogenic factors," and "the transmission of disease in five *zang*-organs." To be specific, "human beings have three excess and three asthenia, i.e., excess and asthenia of pulse, disease and diagnosis ..." (*The Classic of Medical Problems: The 48 Problems*); "pathogenic wind, cold, summer-heat, improper diet and over-work are known as five kinds of pathogenic factors" (*The Classic of Medical Problems: The 49 Problems*); "If the heart disease transmits to the spleen, spleen disease to lungs, lung disease to kidneys, kidney disease to the liver, and liver disease to the heart, this transmission is called 'the disorder of mother organ involving child organ' according to the theory of Five Elements"(*The Classic of Medical Problems: The 53 Problems*).

Moreover, *The Classic of Medical Problems* develops such theories as meridians, *life gate* and pathogenesis of *The Classic of Internal Medicine*, and propounds many important therapeutic principles, such as "reinforcing the mother organ in the treatment of deficiency syndrome and purging the child organ in treating excess syndrome," "strengthening the function of the spleen in the treatment of liver disease, or keeping the spleen off pathogenic factors, for the pathological changes of the liver are likely to transmit to the spleen," and "purging fire and supplementing water" (*The Classic of Medical Problems*).

Obviously, the publication of *The Classic of Medical Problems* and *The Classic of Internal Medicine* shows that medicine is not only a continuation of experiences and practices, but also a theoretical cognition of the cause and law of disease, which symbolizes the establishment of the theoretical system of TCM.

3.2.2 *The Classic of Meteria Medica:* Pharmacological Development

As the first pharmaceutical monograph in China, *The Classic of Meteria Medica* also develops the medical thoughts of *The Classic of Internal Medicine*. The record of Chinese medicinal herbs is no longer the description of the collection, shape and single action, but a comprehensive summary of herbs' grade, taste, nature, property, toxicity, compatibility, collection, preparation, and application. For the first time, it puts forward the basic theories about the compatibility of Chinese medicinal herbs. According to *The Classic of Meteria Medica*, "Chinese medicinal herbs can be divided into monarch herb, minister herb, adjuvant herb and guiding herb in light of their different actions"; "Chinese medicinal herbs have five flavors (sour, salty, sweet, bitter, and pungent), four properties (cold, heat, warm, and cool)"; and "the possible effects of the combination of Chinese medicinal herbs in a prescription are usually called *qiqing.*" The medicinal experiences and the theory of medicinal properties summarized in *The Classic of Meteria Medica* supplement the medication experiences in *The Classic of Internal Medicine* and *The Classic of Medical Problems*, and provide the essential basis for TSD and the application of prescription.

To sum up, the successive publication of *The Classic of Internal Medicine*, *The Classic of Medical Problems*, and *The Classic of Meteria Medica* shows the great achievements in the exploration of disease law and the medication experience accumulation, which symbolizes the establishment of TCM's theoretical system and the standardization of clinical practice.

3.3 Preliminary Establishment of TSD

Treatise on Exogenous Febrile Diseases and Miscellaneous Diseases (the later physicians divide it into two books: *Treatise on Febrile Diseases*[54] and *Synopsis of the Golden Chamber*) establishes the typical model of TSD and integrates medical theory, principle, prescription, and herb for clinical practice. The preliminary establishment of the TSD model is the specific manifestation of the idea of syndrome differentiation advocated in *The Classic of Internal Medicine* in clinical practice. The publication of *Treatise on Exogenous Febrile Diseases and Miscellaneous Diseases* symbolizes the great reform of medical practice from intuitionistic experience into theory-instructed experience.

The Treatise on Febrile Diseases distinguishes the concepts of disease and syndrome.

The concept of disease in *Treatise on Febrile Diseases* is not a complete process including specific etiology, the form of onset, pathogenesis, development and prognosis, but a generalization of pathological manifestations of a certain kind of pathological phenomenon. There are six diseases in *Treatise on Febrile Diseases*: *taiyang* disease, *yangming* disease, *shaoyang* disease, *taiyin* disease, *shaoyin* disease, and *jueyin* disease. "*Taiyang* disease is manifested as floating pulse, stiffness and pain of head and neck, and aversion to cold"; "*Yangming* disease is manifested as high fever, polydipsia, polyhidrosis, full and large pulse, constipation and abdominal pain"; "*Shaoyang* disease is manifested as bitter taste in mouth, dry throat and dizziness"; "*Taiyin* disease is manifested as abdominal distension and even vomiting, inability to get food down, diarrhea and abdominal pain"; "*Shaoyin* disease is manifested as faint and thin pulse and sleepiness"; and "*Jueyin* disease is manifested as polydipsia, polyuria, hunger without appetite, and incessant diarrhea if treating it with purgative therapy."

Syndrome, according to *Treatise on Febrile Diseases*, is the combination of symptoms reflecting the essence of a certain disease. It can be divided into two categories: syndrome of disease and syndrome of prescription. The former refers to the pathological stage of a certain disease, e.g., "for *taiyang* disease, if the syndrome is of such clinical manifestations as fever, sweating, aversion to wind and floating pulse, it is called wind-attack syndrome of *taiyang* disease" and "if the syndrome is of such clinical manifestations as aversion to cold, pain in limbs, vomiting and tight pulse, it is cold-attack syndrome of *taiyang* disease." The second category, the syndrome of prescription, refers to the syndrome that a certain prescription is mainly targeted at, e.g., "the syndrome with such clinical manifestations as floating and slow pulse, exterior heat and interior cold, as well as diarrhea with undigested food should be treated with *Sini Tang* (Decoction for Resuscitation), and is called the syndrome of *Sini Tang* (Decoction for Resuscitation)" and "The syndrome with such clinical manifestations as floating pulse, fever, dry mouth with desire for drink and dysuria should be treated with *Zhuling Tang* (Umbellate Pore Decoction), and is known as the syndrome of *Zhuling Tang* (Umbellate Pore Decoction)."

Treatise on Febrile Diseases records more than thirty kinds of syndromes of disease (such as cold-attack syndrome, wind-attack syndrome, cold-attack syndrome, syndrome of blood accumulation, and syndrome of yang exhaustion), and 113 kinds of syndromes of prescription (such as the syndrome of *Guizhi Tang*, the syndrome of *Baihu Tang*, and the syndrome of *Chaihu Tang*). Syndrome is the key of TSD for any disease, even for the complicated disease involving two or three meridians. For example, "*Taiyang* disease, manifested as stiffness of nape and back, absence of sweating, and aversion to wind, should be treated with *Gegen Tang*," "the disease involving both *taiyang* and *yangming* manifested as absence of sweating, aversion to wind and diarrhea, should be treated with *Gegen Tang*" and "the disease involving both *taiyang* and *yangming* manifested as dyspnea and fullness in chest should be treated not with purgation but with *Mahuang Tang*." These show that the same disease with different syndromes should be treated with different therapeutic methods and different diseases with the same syndrome should be treated with the same therapeutic method. Therefore, syndrome is the basis to decide the therapeutic methods. It is not the simple combination of symptoms, but the essence of disease. Although the theoretical cognition of syndrome has not yet been proposed at that time, medical treatment has been made based on syndrome differentiation in practice.

In addition, *Treatise on Febrile Diseases* has already standardized 150 symptoms, including thirty kinds of general symptoms (such as fever, aversion to wind, sweating, spontaneous sweating, jaundice, and arthralgia of limbs), twenty kinds of head symptoms (such as headache, dizziness, bitter taste in the mouth, red eyes, and dryness of nose), ten kinds of symptoms of four limbs (such as cold limbs, cold extremities, and spasm), sixty kinds of visceral symptoms (like restlessness, insomnia, palpitation due to fright, murmuring in an unconscious state, hiccup, vomiting, diarrhea, and dysuria), twenty kinds of symptoms of chest and abdomen (like fullness in the chest and hypochondrium, hypochondriac fullness and rigidity, abdominal pain, abdominal distention and fullness, epigastric stuffiness and pain, pain and heat in the heart, hypochondriac pain and lump), and twenty kinds of pulse conditions (such as floating pulse, sunken pulse, rapid pulse as well as knotted pulse, and slow-regular-intermittent pulse). Some common symptoms appear many times in the book and some only once or twice. For example, "fever" appears more than one hundred times in *Treatise on Febrile Diseases*, e.g., "in *taiyang* disease, the syndrome with such clinical manifestations as fever, sweating, aversion to wind and floating pulse is called wind-attack syndrome of *taiyang* disease" and "if patients who just suffer from *shaoyang* disease have fever and sunken pulse, they should be treated with *Mahuang Fuzi Xixin Tang*"; "aversion to cold" and "sweating" both appear more than seventy times; as for "headache," "aversion to cold" and "alternate attack of chills and fever" and other symptoms, some symptoms appear dozens of times and some only more than ten times. Analyzing these common exogenous symptoms that repeatedly appear, we can generalize the law of these symptoms and their combination with other symptoms. It is the content of syndrome differentiation.

Only when the law of syndrome variation is grasped, can treatment be made based on syndrome differentiation. As to syndrome differentiation of "sweating" and "no sweating," for instance, "*Taiyang* disease that is manifested as headache, fever, sweating and aversion to wind should be treated with *Guizhi Tang*," "after treated with the method of diaphoresis, if patients who suffer from *Taiyang* disease have such symptoms as aversion to wind, dysuria and spasm of limbs, they should be treated with *Guizhi Jia Fuzi Tang*," "*Taiyang* disease that is manifested as headache, fever, lumbago, arthralgia, aversion to wind, no sweating and dyspnea should be treated with *Mahuang Tang*" and "*Taiyang* disease which is manifested as stiffness of nape and back, absence of sweating and aversion to wind should be treated with *Gegen Tang*." All of them show that the exterior syndrome with sweating should be treated with *Guizhi Tang* Serial Decoctions and the exterior syndrome with no sweating should be treated with *Mahuang Tang* Serial Decoctions.

The precise differentiation of primary symptoms in *Treatise on Febrile Diseases* shows that at that time ancient Chinese have learned a lot about the relationship between prescription and syndrome.

To reflect the essence of syndrome, treatment should be done on the differentiation between primary symptoms and secondary symptoms, as well as their laws of variation. For example, "fever with no sweating" and "fever with sweating" have the same primary symptom of "fever," but the essences of syndromes are different in secondary symptoms concerning "sweating," and therefore their therapeutic methods are different. The former is treated using *Mahuang Tang* with *Herba Ephedrae* (Chinese ephedra herb) as monarch herb, and the latter using *Guizhi Tang* with *Ramulus Cinnamomi* as monarch herb. These therapeutic practices based on prescription-syndrome relation are distinct from previous practices based on drug-symptom relation, though the former relies on the latter. It can be expounded with the difference between herbs in the principal prescription and those in the class prescription. For example, among six kinds of *Mahuang Tang* Serial Decoctions, *Mahuang Tang* is the principal prescription and *Da Qinglong Tang* is one of its class prescriptions. The syndromes treated with *Mahuang Tang* are headache, fever, lumbago, arthralgia, aversion to wind, no sweating and dyspnea; the syndromes treated with *Da Qinglong Tang* are floating and tight pulse, fever, aversion to cold, general pain, no sweating and dysphoria. The symptoms listed above are similar, but the symptom of dysphoria only appears in the syndrome of *Da Qinglong Tang*, so *Da Qinglong Tang* is composed of *Mahuang Tang* and *Gypsum Fibrosum*, which can cure dysphoria.

Based on such drug-symptom practices, prescription-syndrome experiences are highly summarized and taken as guidelines in therapeutic activities. For example, the therapeutic method of diaphoresis is applied according to the prescription inducing sweating or reducing the exterior syndrome. And the therapeutic method of purgation is applied according to the prescription promoting purgation.

In *Treatise on Febrile Diseases*, 113 prescriptions made up of more than eighty kinds of Chinese medicinal herbs are summarized to correspond with eight basic therapeutic methods: diaphoresis, emesis, purgation, regulating therapy, warming therapy, cooling therapy, supplementing, or resolving therapy. Thus, the typical model of TSD is preliminarily established.

The other essential part of *Treatise on Exogenous Febrile Diseases and Miscellaneous Diseases*, *Synopsis of the Golden Chamber* elaborates TSD, focusing on the cognition and the treatment of miscellaneous diseases due to the internal damages.

First, to make disease differentiation and syndrome differentiation, *Synopsis of the Golden Chamber* categorizes diseases in terms of primary symptoms. Such a perspective can be seen from the names of chapters of the book, such as "Treatment of Hemiplegia and Arthralgia Firstly Based on Disease Differentiation and then on Syndrome Differentiation" and "Treatment of Thoracic Obstruction and Precordial Pain Firstly Based on Disease Differentiation and Then on Syndrome Differentiation." *Synopsis of the Golden Chamber* has twenty-five chapters and more than 400 items about syndrome differentiation, in which more than forty kinds of diseases and 262 prescriptions are recorded.

Second, the prescriptions that are used to treat exogenous febrile diseases in *Treatise on Febrile Diseases* are applied to treat the internal damages and other diseases in *Synopsis of the Golden Chamber*, e.g., *Guizhi Tang* Serial Decoctions. It shows the flexibility of TSD.

Third, *Synopsis of the Golden Chamber* accumulates rich medication experiences based on symptoms to treat miscellaneous diseases due to internal damages. For example, as for thoracic obstruction, primary symptoms like pain in the chest are treated with *Fructus Trichosanthis* and *Bulbus Allii Macrostemi*. As to its secondary symptoms like vomiting, *Rhizoma Pinelliae* is added to the above herbs, and if a secondary symptom is abdominal distention, *Fructus Aurantii Immaturus* and *Cortex Magnoliae Officinalis* are added.

Treatise on Febrile Diseases summarizes the law of TSD in treating exogenous febrile diseases, and *Synopsis of the Golden Chamber* accumulates the rich medication experiences in treating miscellaneous diseases due to internal damages, and thus the publication of *Treatise on Exogenous Febrile Diseases and Miscellaneous Diseases* symbolizes the establishment of the TSD model.

3.4 Accumulation of Therapeutic Experiences

After the establishment of the TSD model in *Treatise on Exogenous Febrile Diseases and Miscellaneous Diseases*, the ancient experiential medicine gradually got mature.

The Jin dynasty (265–420 A.D.) and the Tang dynasty (618–907 A.D.) are the times when TCM's clinical practice was fully developed. For one thing, the previous medical theories and clinical experiences were collected and interpreted. For example, *Plain Questions* was annotated by Quan Yuanqi in the Sui dynasty, Yang Shangshan[55] in the Sui and Tang dynasties, and commented by Wang Bing.[56] *Treatise on Febrile Diseases* was reorganized by Wang Shuhe.[57] For another, sphygmology, etiology, pharmacology, and clinical branches have advanced a lot. A large number of relevant works appeared, exerting great influence on the later clinical medicine, such as *A Handbook of Prescriptions for Emergencies*, *The General Treatise on the Etiology and Symptomatology of Diseases*, *The Essential Remedies*,[58] and *Medical Secrets of an Official*.

3.4.1 Furthering Cognition of Disease

First, based on *The Classic of Internal Medicine*, *The Classic of Medical Problems*, and *Treatise on Febrile Diseases*, Wang Shuhe, in volume 6 of *The Pulse Classic*, developed the theory of visceral pathogenesis. He takes *zang-fu* organs as outline and asthenia-excess as item, analyzing the occurrence, transmission, and clinical manifestation of diseases and pathological changes of emotion and meridians-collaterals. And it is the inchoate theory of visceral pathogenesis.

Second, Chao Yuanfang[59] put forward many new understandings of etiology, and pathogenesis in *The General Treatise on the Etiology and Symptomatology of Diseases*. This book elaborates diseases of thirty-nine branches like internal medicine, surgery, gynecology, pediatrics, ophthalmology, dermatology, and otorhinolaryngology, and 1, 739 kinds of syndromes such as apoplexy, wind stroke, and trismus. It comprehensively elaborates the cause and pathogenesis of each kind of disease based on *The Classic of Internal Medicine*. For example, "as for the syndrome of paralysis due to the attack of wind, its cause and pathogenesis is that patients' muscular interstices are open out of the deficiency of *qi* and blood, and when they are attacked by pathogenic wind, their muscles cannot be nourished by blood due to blood stagnation, and finally paralysis appears." Besides, there are many etiological breakthroughs in *The General Treatise on the Etiology and Symptomatology of Diseases*, for instance, Chao Yuanfang found that scabies was a contagious skin disease caused by the itch mite, and pestilence had strong infectivity and was easy to spread.

Third, in the annotation of *Plain Questions*, Wang Bing also expounded his viewpoint in pathogenesis and generalized the causes and pathogenesis of diseases into four categories: "internal diseases with lesions of organs caused by the changes of visceral *qi*, like abdominal mass and tuberculosis; external diseases with lesions of superficial tissues, such as carbuncle and tumefaction; internal disorders due to changes of visceral *qi*, like dyspepsia and melancholia; and external disorders due to external injury, such as puncture wound as well as insect and animal bite."

Fourth, *The Essential Remedies*, a great medical masterpiece integrating internal medicine, surgery, gynecology, diet therapy, health maintenance, herbs, prescription and medical ethic, developed the theoretical cognition of syndrome. It differentiates symptoms of visceral diseases and generalizes symptoms into cold, heat, excess and asthenia, and it also brings forward the notions of syndrome, such as "sthenia-heat syndrome of liver," "excess-heat syndrome of gallbladder," "asthenia-cold syndrome of liver", and "asthenia-cold syndrome of gallbladder." It is the earliest theoretical cognition of syndrome differentiation of viscera, and exerts great influence on the theoretical perfection of TSD.

3.4.2 Improving Therapeutic Understanding

The development of clinical medicine in the Jin and Tang dynasties is mainly embodied in the enrichment of practical experiences and constant emergence of the medical formularies, like *Yu Han Fang*[60] and *A Handbook of Prescriptions for Emergencies* written by Ge Hong,[61] *Jotting Prescriptions*[62] by Chen Yanzhi, *The Essential Remedies* and *The Supplement Remedies*[63] by Sun Simiao, *A Collection of Effective Recipes*[64] by Yao Sengyuan, and *Medical Secrets of an Official* by Wang Tao.[65] Unfortunately, only several books remain now, such as *A Handbook of Prescriptions for Emergencies*, *The Essential Remedies*, and *Medical Secrets of an Official*.

Treatise on Febrile Diseases was not popular in the Jin and Tang dynasties, so there was no medical formulary that inherited the system of TSD comprehensively. Only a few therapeutic experiences were kept in some medical formularies, in which the most important ones were *A Collection of Effective Recipes* and *Jotting Prescriptions*. *A Collection of Effective*

Recipes names every chapter as "Prescriptions Used to Treat XX Disease or XX Syndrome" (such as "Prescriptions Used to Treat Exogenous Febrile Diseases"), and involves diseases of internal medicine, surgery, gynecology, pediatrics, ophthalmology, and otorhinolaryngology. Its description of the syndrome of prescription is similar to that of *Treatise on Febrile Diseases*. The difference is that the laws of prescription application and laws of syndrome change are not clearly stated in *A Collection of Effective Recipes*. The contents and characteristics of *Jotting Prescriptions* are the same as those of *A Collection of Effective Recipes*. It shows that *Jotting Prescriptions* and *A Collection of Effective Recipes* all record simple therapeutic experiences.

The Essential Remedies written by Sun Simiao in the Tang dynasty develops the contents of TSD in *Treatise on Febrile Diseases*, and propels the medication of that time. It has embodied the explicit feature of "syndrome differentiation of viscera." As to excess-heat syndrome of lungs, for example, it not only covers the differentiation of symptoms (e.g., cough and red tongue with yellowish fur are clinical manifestations of excess-heat syndrome of lung, while cough and reddish tongue with little fur are symptoms of asthenia-heat syndrome of lung), but also involves the corresponding therapeutic prescription, namely, *Weijing Tang* (Reed Stem Decoction). Along with *The Essential Remedies*, *Medical Secrets of an Office* complied by Wang Tao, another medical masterpiece in the Tang dynasty, furthered the practical model of TSD and made it widely used in medical practice.

3.5 Theory Inheritance and Practice Standardization

From the Jin and Tang dynasties to the middle period of the Northern Song dynasty, the theoretical cognition of TSD was still the syndrome differentiation of visceral diseases. And the mainstream of clinical medicine was still the application and accumulation of therapeutic experiences. Abundant as practical experiences are, TSD still needs theoretical summarization.

The Song, Jin, and Yuan dynasties are critical turning points in the history of TCM. Medical practitioners of various schools expound their own medical theories according to their own clinical experiences, promoting the perfection of theoretical exploration.

First, physicians in the Song, Jin, and Yuan dynasties studied and annotated many ancient medical works, especially the *Treatise on Febrile Diseases*. The most famous annotators and their works are as follows: in the Song dynasty, *Febrile Diseases Note* (by Cheng Wuji),[66] *On Febrile Diseases* (by Pang Anshi), *Profound Comments on Febrile Diseases* (by Han Zhihe), *A Classified Book on Treating Febrile Diseases* (by Zhu Gong), *Expounding Febrile Diseases* (by Xu Shuwei), *Addendum to Treatise on Febrile Diseases* (by Guo Yong) and *General Treatise on Febrile Diseases* (by Yang Shiying); in the Jin and Yuan dynasties, they are *The Essentials of the Treatment of Febrile* (by Liu Hong), *Differentiation of Febrile Diseases*[67] (by Ma Zongsu), and so on. They all emphasize the study of TSD in the *Treatise on Febrile Diseases*, but differ in their perspectives. For example, Cheng Wuji turned to *The Classic of Internal Medicine* to annotate the *Treatise on Febrile Diseases*; Zhu Gong turned to *yin* and *yang* to differentiate syndromes in treating exogenous febrile diseases; Xu Shuwei pointed out that exogenous febrile diseases should be treated based on the differentiation of external syndrome and internal syndrome, as well as asthenia syndrome and excess syndrome; Liu Wansu brought forward that febrile diseases should be treated on the basis of the differentiation of cold syndrome and heat syndrome.

In fact, the annotation of *Treatise on Febrile Diseases* and the theoretical generalization of external syndrome and internal syndrome, *yin* syndrome and *yang* syndrome, cold syndrome and heat syndrome as well as asthenia syndrome and excess syndrome, all based theories on *The Classic of Internal Medicine*. In the Song, Jin, and Yuan dynasties, physicians provided the theoretical basis for TSD with etiology and pathogenesis in *The Classic of Internal*

Medicine. Under the influence of this thought, physicians shifted their academic interest from medication practice to theoretical reflection and many theories appeared, e.g., the theory of "Three Types of Etiologic Factors" by Chen Wuze, the theory of "eliminating pathogenic factors" by Zhang Congzheng, and the theory of "nourishing yin" by Zhu Zhenheng. So TSD in this period focuses on the theoretical establishment of "syndrome," rather than on the summarization of therapeutic experiences. And the clinical treatment focuses on the differentiation of the nature of a disease such as cold and heat, external and internal, as well as asthenia and excess, rather than on the differentiation of complicated symptoms. And thus the "syndrome" of TSD is theoretically established. The establishment of the TSD system in the Song, Jin, and Yuan dynasties symbolized the final unification of theory and practice of TCM.

3.6 Complete Summary of Clinical Experiences and the Perfection of the TSD Model

The unity of theory and practice was completed in the Song, Jin, and Yuan dynasties. After the Ming and Qing dynasties, TCM's academic system was further perfected with the incorporation of theories like life-gate, *xianghuo*, *triple energizer*, and seasonal febrile diseases. In clinical practice, TSD has become a basic principle. The guiding principle of syndrome differentiation of various diseases is "syndrome differentiation with eight principles." That is, syndromes are usually differentiated from the aspects of *yin* and *yang*, external and internal, cold and heat, as well as asthenia and exces.

The final establishment of TSD promoted the standardization of clinical practice in the Ming and Qing dynasties. Up to 1950s, with the rise of TCM education, scholars of TCM comprehensively and systematically summarized the basic ideas, principles, contents, and methods of TSD, and further standardized the names of syndromes, which made TSD more concrete and applicable. With reference to Jia Dedao's *A General History of Traditional Chinese Medicine*, we summarize the principles of TSD as follows:

Principle 1: Make every effort to differentiate the nature of disease.
> Maxim 1: Try to differentiate the syndrome of asthenia and excess as well as cold and heat. (This is the basic form of the change of disease.)
> Maxim 2: Try to differentiate *six excesses* (wind, cold, summer-heat, dampness, dryness, and heat) and *seven emotions* (terror, anxiety, anger, contemplation, grief, fear, and joy). (This is the differentiation of the causes of disease.)
> Maxim 3: Try to differentiate the syndromes of *yin* and *yang*. (This is the basic principle of syndrome differentiation.)

Principle 2: Spare no effort to differentiate the location of disease.
> Maxim 1: Try to differentiate external and internal.
> Maxim 2: Try to differentiate the *zang* organ and *fu* organ.
> Maxim 3: Try to differentiate meridians and collaterals.
> Maxim 4: Try to differentiate *qi*, blood, and body fluid.
> Maxim 5: Try to differentiate defensive phase, *qi* phase, nutrient phase, and blood phase.
> Maxim 6: Try to differentiate *triple energizer*.

After a long-term accumulation of practical experiences, theoretical reflection, and medical standardization, TSD has developed into an effective guideline for TCM's clinical practice.

CHAPTER 4
Basic Features of TCM

Objectives & Requirements
1. Basic features of TCM.
2. Definition and connotation of the holism view of TCM.
3. Organic integrity of the human body.
4. Unity of man and nature.
5. Definition and connotation of TSD.
6. Definitions and the distinction of symptom, syndrome, and disease.
7. Main content of syndrome differentiation.
8. Main content of TCM's treatment.
9. Relation between syndrome differentiation and treatment.
10. Principles of TSD.

Key Concepts
1. Two characteristics peculiar to TCM are holism and TSD.
2. Holism is an important concept of TCM. It refers to both the integrity of the human body itself, and the unity of the human body and nature. As an organic integrity, different parts of the human body are inseparable in structure, coordinative in physiology, and mutually interacting in pathology. Meanwhile, the unity of the human body and nature lies in the fact that the human body is influenced by the natural conditions, and therefore human beings have to adapt to nature to maintain their normal vital activities.
3. The human body is regarded as an organic integrity in terms of the following three aspects: the integrity of man's physical structure, the unity of its various physiological functions, as well as the unity of structures and their functions. The local and the whole of the human body are correlated in pathological changes, and therefore the wholeness should be taken into great consideration in the processes of diagnosis, treatment, and health maintenance.
4. The unity of man and nature can be expounded from the natural and social impacts on man's physiological activities. The former mainly refers to the influence of climate and geographic environment on the human body. As to the latter, the progress, peace, or turmoil of the society as well as the change of individual's social status are the most important factors affecting one's physiological functions.
5. TSD, as a fundamental feature of TCM, is also the basic principle of disease identification and treatment in TCM. Syndrome differentiation means to analyze the data collected through inspection, auscultation and olfaction, interrogation, as well as pulse taking and palpation, so as to understand the cause, nature, and location of disease, as well as the relationship between pathogenic factors and vital energy, and finally make a diagnosis of syndrome. Treatment here means to decide the therapeutic methods according to the result of syndrome differentiation.
6. To understand the concept of syndrome, a comparison must be made between disease, syndrome, and symptom. Disease is a complete process including the specific etiology, the form of onset, pathogenesis, development, and prognosis. Symptoms are the concrete clinical manifestations. Syndrome is a summary of pathological changes

of a disease at a certain stage in the course of its development, involving the cause, location, and nature of disease, as well as the relationship of pathogenic factors and vital energy.

7. Syndrome differentiation involves the differentiations of symptoms and signs, etiology and pathogenesis, location, nature, state and tendency, superficiality and origin, and the pattern of disease. From different perspectives, they are interrelated in reflecting the nature and the intrinsic relation of diseases.
8. Treatment involves determining therapeutic methods and measures, deciding prescriptions, and performing the treatment.
9. The relationship between syndrome differentiation and treatment goes as follows: the former is the prerequisite to the latter, while the latter is the aim of the former. The curative effect is the test to the syndrome differentiation and treatment.
10. Four principles of TSD are TSD should (1) be guided by the concept of holism; (2) follow the law of syndrome; (3) combine syndrome differentiation with disease differentiation; (4) make necessary adaptation while abiding by the above principles.

The theoretical system of TCM has been gradually formed in the long history of clinical practice under the guidance of ancient materialism and dialectic. Its distinctive characteristics are the concepts of holism and TSD.

4.1 The Concept of Holism

Holism is an important concept of TCM. It refers to the integrity of the human body itself and the unity of the human body and nature as well. As an organic integrity, parts of the human body are inseparable in structure, coordinative in physiology, and mutually interacting in pathology. Meanwhile, the unity of the human body and nature lies in the fact that the human body is influenced by the natural conditions and therefore human beings have to adapt to nature to maintain their normal vital activities. This notion was the manifestation of ancient materialism and dialectic, permeating such TCM aspects as physiology, pathology, diagnostic methods, syndrome differentiation, and treatment.

4.1.1 The Human Body: An Organic Integrity

The human body is an organic integrity in the following three aspects. As far as structure is concerned, it is composed of various organs and tissues which are not only closely related, but also indispensable to the whole. Concerning building substance, its integrity lies in the fact that its *zang-fu* organs and their functions are exclusively composed of and supported by such substances as essence, *qi* (vital energy), blood, and body fluids. These substances distribute and circulate in the whole body, carrying out various functional activities. Besides, it is in their functional activities that the human body is also integrated, i.e., due to the wholeness of the structure and the substantiality of building substances, various functional activities are not only interdependent but also mutually interacting, not only coordinative but also mutually restricting.

4.1.1.1 The Integrity of Physical Structures

The related and inseparable components of the human body are head, face, four limbs, meridians, and trunk, as the well as internal five *zang*-organs (a collective term for heart, liver, spleen, lung and kidney), six *fu*-organs (a collective term for gallbladder, stomach, small intestine, large intestine, *triple energizer*, and the urinary bladder), extraordinary *fu*-organs (a collective term for brain, marrow, bones, vessels, gallbladder, and uterus), and *qi*, blood, and various body fluids. The unity of the human body, according to the theory of TCM, is realized through the dominant role of five *zang*-organs, the assistance of six *fu*-organs, and the function of the meridian system internally pertaining to viscera and externally connecting limbs.

- **Physical Integrity Centering Around Five *Zang*-Organs**

In terms of TCM, various *zang-fu* organs, sensory organs, orifices, five constituents (tendons, vessels, muscles, skin, bones, etc.), four limbs, and all skeletal parts, are not only directly related to one another in structure, but also indirectly linked centering around five *zang*-organs through the meridian system. The significant role of five *zang*-organs in the unity of physical structure lies in the fact that they, with their corresponding *fu*-organs, constituents, sensory organs, orifices, limbs, and joints, form five important functional systems. The liver system is dominated by the liver, assisted by the gallbladder, and associated with eyes, tendons, hands, etc.; the heart system takes the heart as the main part, pertains to the small intestine, and associates with tongue, face, vessels, etc.; the spleen system takes the spleen as the leader, pertains to the stomach, and associates with lips, mouth, muscles, limbs, etc.; the lung system, led by lungs, pertains to the large intestine, and associates with nose, skin, and hairs etc.; the kidney system, dominated by kidneys, pertains to urinary bladder, and associates with ears, hairs, bones, external genitalia, anus, etc. Every local part of each system is the constituent of the whole body, based on traditional Chinese *yin-yang* and Five Elements.

- **Physical Integrity Bridged by the Meridian System**

The meridian system, including meridians, collaterals, and their related parts, functions as a channel where *qi* and blood circulate. It is also a network where viscera, sensory organs, orifices, skin, five constituents, four limbs, and all the skeletal parts are connected.

The meridian system is an important component of the human body, for the dynamic connection and structural integrity of the human body are realized not only by the direct connection between viscera and other organs, but also by the indirect link via meridians and collaterals. For example, the important *Twelve Meridians* of the human body are divided into two categories: *yin* meridians and *yang* meridians. The former pertain to *zang*-organs and connect *fu*-organs, while the latter are the opposite. Like *zang*-organs and *fu*-organs, they form an internal-external pair, allowing *qi* and blood to infuse through the connected channels. The indivisible meridian system is carried on with *yin* meridians and *yang* meridians connecting with each other following a certain circulating and infusing order, and at the same time eight extra meridians, tendons of twelve meridians, fifteen main collaterals, and twelve cutaneous regions also link each other by *qi* and blood.

4.1.1.2 The Unity of Physiological Functions

The normal performance of organic activities first depends on the regular work of respective viscera and tissues, neither excessively nor deficiently, and then relies on their coordination, either assisting or restricting each other. Every viscus or tissue has to work independently as an individual and dependently as a whole, which demonstrates another sense of unity: local and whole.

For one thing, centering around five *zang*-organs, five functional systems work individually. The heart system, with the heart as the leader, transports *qi* and blood, governs the mind, and regulates the whole body. When the heart system works well, we are healthy with organs and tissues functioning harmoniously. The liver is the dominant part of the liver system, whose function is to govern *shu xie* (dredging the routes and regulating the movement of *qi*), store blood and regulate the circulation of *qi* and blood, and protect the body against pathogenic factors. The spleen system, with the spleen at the core, transports and transforms food into nutrients, enhancing the vital energy of the human body against pathogenic factors and their harmful result. The lung system, dominated by the lungs, regulates the functional activities of the human body by taking charge of the production and transportation of *qi* throughout the whole body. The kidney system, with the dominance of the kidneys, stores essence, and governs reproduction, *qi*-transformation (changes caused by the movement of *qi*), external genitals and the anus, and excretion. Among the five systems, the heart system plays a dominant role in integrating and coordinating other systems. *The Classic of Internal Medicine* makes an analogy: as the safety of a country depends on the wise leadership of a monarch, the normal function of viscera depends on the forceful dominance of the heart; a fragile heart, like a brittle monarch, is incapable of guaranteeing the coordination of viscera.

For another, different as they are in structure and function, the five systems mutually influence each other based on the interrelationship of *zang-xiang* (viscera and their manifestation). The complicated relationship can be accounted for in terms of such principles of *yin-yang* and Five Elements as "to keep *yin-yang* balance," "harm of hyperactivity," and "interrestriction yielding generation and transformation." They can explain how *zang*-organs and *fu*-organs mutually restrict, promote, and transform, and thus keep the whole body in a stable condition of generation and transformation.

4.1.1.3   The Unity of the Human Body's Structure and Function

The integrity of various physical structures and the consubstantiality of building substances determine the coordination and inseparability of the human body's structure and function. It can be explained with the theories of *yin-yang* and Five Elements, which stress the unity of *zang* and *xiang*, the connection of body and spirit, and the correlation between viscera and the meridian system.

Zang-xiang theory investigates the relationship between the human body's structure and function, by dividing the life phenomenon into two basic levels: *zang* and *xiang*. The former pertains to *yin*, and collectively refers to the internal viscera and tissues, as well as their functions and changes, which cannot be directly observed by the eyes. On the contrary, the latter pertains to *yang*, and refers to those observable external organs and tissues, as well as their functions and changes. *Zang-xiang* theory is the high generalization of *qi*-transforming activity, physical structures, and pathological changes caused by the interaction of *yin* and *yang*. Because of the inside-outside correspondence between *zang* and *xiang*, internal physiological and pathological changes manifest themselves as the superficial features of the human body, which help us deduce the internal diseases. This method is called "Judging the Interior from the Exterior Manifestations."

The unity of the human body's structure and function can also be illustrated in the relationship between body and spirit, the two major elements of the life process. They form a type of structure-function relation: inter-depending, interpromoting, and inter-restricting. According to TCM, a human's mental activities can be generalized as spirit, ethereal soul, corporeal soul, mind and will, which are respectively generated and governed by the heart, the liver, lungs, the spleen, kidneys, and reflect seven types of emotion: joy, anger, anxiety, contemplation, grief, terror, and fear. Namely, "the five *zang*-organs dominate five kinds of visceral *qi* to produce various emotions" (*Plain Questions*, Chapter 5). Mental activities, produced in organic process, govern physical organism, and therefore the "maintenance of spirit ensures life, while loss of spirit causes death" (*Plain Questions*, Chapter 13), for "the loss of spirit will sever the mechanism of generation and transformation" (*Plain Questions*, Chapter 70). TCM emphasizes the coexistence of body and spirit in the maintenance of normal vital activities: "body is the basis of spirit, and spirit is the function of body. Body lives on spirit, and spirit lives in body" (*Classified Canon*,[68] Chapter 19).

Besides, the unity of the human body's structure and function can also be interpreted into the correlation between viscera and the meridian system. The human body's organic activities depend on an integral organism with five *zang*-organs at the center, with meridians and collaterals as a bridge between internal *zang-fu* organs and external limbs, joints, and orifices, and supported by essence, *qi*, blood and body fluids in meridians and collaterals, which are not only the building materials of an organism, but also the energy sources for various functional activities. In this way, the whole body is unified.

4.1.1.4 Local-Whole Relationship in Pathological Changes

Under the guidance of holism, TCM also probes into the law of pathogenesis. Namely, in TCM, a diagnosis is made from an integral perspective. In the analysis of local lesions, their direct relation with corresponding viscera, and indirect relation with other viscera are taken into much consideration. For one thing, any local lesion is the manifestation of, and maybe the reason for, some visceral disease. For example, dryness of the eyes can be the manifestation of the insufficiency of liver-*yin* and liver-blood, for the liver is closely related to the eyes. For another, pathological changes of different viscera are mutually influential. A good case in point is that the deficiency of kidney-*yin* may result in the insufficiency of liver-*yin*, and the prolonged deficiency of liver-blood can lead to the inadequacy of kidney-*yin*. The reason is that the liver and kidneys are so close to each other that they are believed to "share the same origin"; kidney-*yin* is the source of liver-*yin*, and liver-blood is the material for liver-*yin* to nurture kidney-*yin*.

Diseases can be distinguished as local or whole, due to their location, duration, and the seriousness of the injury to the vital energy. Therefore, in diagnosis, importance should be attached to the wholeness of the syndrome, as well as the relation between the local pathological changes and the whole pathological conditions. For example, the whole pathological changes caused by "the failure to control blood and fluid due to *qi* deficiency" may lead to various local illnesses such as hemorrhagic syndrome (epistaxis, hematohidrosis, metrorrhagia, and metrostaxis), seminal emission, diarrhea, proctoptosis, and so on. The local carbuncle and sores, if not treated promptly and properly, will cause the disorder of meridians and five *zang*-organs, even death. It reveals the law of diseases, i.e., the local and whole diseases are mutually influential and constantly change in the process of pathological development.

4.1.1.5 Local-Whole Relationship in Diagnosis

Local and whole form a dialectical unity in that the local pathological changes are often related to the conditions of viscera, *qi* and blood, as well as *yin* and *yang* of the whole body. Owing to the interrelation and interaction of various physiological functions and pathological changes, internal pathological changes can express themselves as the external features in such aspects as five sense organs, physique, complexion, and pulse. These aspects enable us to understand and judge visceral diseases, and make correct diagnoses and treatments.

The observation of complexion and tongue is an important part of inspection, one important diagnostic method in TCM. It is believed that the facial color and luster are the signs of *qi* and blood in viscera, because first "*qi* originates from viscera, and face with luster is the manifestation of *qi* sufficiency" (*Essentials for Four Diagnosis*)[69], and second "the circulation of *qi* and blood in twelve channels and three hundred and sixty five collaterals reach the face first, and then enter various apertures" (*Spiritual Pivot*, Chapter 4). It shows that complex ion is the manifestation of the conditions of the heart and other viscera, whose essence reaches the face through meridians. Consequently, the observation of facial color and luster can tell us the conditions of *qi* and blood in viscera as well as the location of pathogenic factors.

Tongue observation is another essential approach to inspecting the functional states of viscera, because the tongue connects with five *zang*-organs directly or indirectly through meridians. "The heart opens into tongue, and other four *zang*-organs connect with the heart through meridians which all reach tongue." Therefore, the state of the tongue can reflect the physiological functions and pathological changes of viscera and meridians. Observing the tongue is a reliable way to differentiate syndromes of asthenia and excess, *yin* and *yang*, as well as *zang* and *fu* (*Diagnostic Method Depending on Tongue Inspection*).[70]

Pulse-taking, one important part of pulse-feeling and palpation, is another effective way to diagnose the condition of inner viscera, for the pulse condition is in close relation to the circulation of *qi* and blood in viscera, which may be affected by the working state of viscera themselves. Specifically, the heart dominates blood generation, lungs control blood circulation, the spleen and stomach are the source of *qi* and blood (the spleen also keeps the blood flowing), the liver stores blood, and kidneys store essence (the source of *yang-qi* and one essential material foundation of blood production). Therefore, the disorder of any viscera will affect the circulation of *qi* and blood, and thus manifest itself in the pulse condition, through which we can judge the location and infer the prognosis of disease.

Holism, the important concept of TCM, has also been proved in other fields. Modern biological holography shows that certain local changes of the organism can reflect the internal and overall conditions of the human body to a considerable extent. Under the guidance of holism, the ancient Chinese medical scientists created and developed a series of methods and theories. According to them, the conditions of viscera and the whole body can be observed through the changes of tongue, pulse, and some parts of body surface.

4.1.1.6 The Wholeness of the Therapeutic Process

Like diagnosis, the treatment of diseases is also guided by holism. First, the concept of holism can be applied to the treatment of local lesions because of the close relation between *zang*-organs, *fu*-organs, configurations, and orifices. For example, ophthalmic diseases are often cured with the same method to treat liver diseases, for the liver opens into the eyes. Another example is that sores in the mouth are cured by purging excess heat in the heart and small intestine, for the heart, which is internally and externally related to the small intestine, opens into the tongue.

Second, diseases of the five *zang*-organs are treated integrally because the disorder of one organ may be transmitted to another for their intrinsic interrelation. For example, "measures must be taken to strengthen the function of the spleen in the treatment of liver disease, or to keep spleen off pathogenic factors," for "the pathological changes of the liver is much likely to transmit to the spleen." "Such a therapeutic method is called treating disease before its onset" (*Classic of Medical Problems*). The method, deducing the development of disease and determining therapeutic strategies based on the relationship between the five *zang*-organs, is the specific application of holism in treatment.

Third, holism is also applied to acupuncture and moxibustion therapies. For example, "pathogenic factors in *yang* meridians can be cured by acupuncturing *yin* meridians, and vice versa. Likewise, diseases on the left sides can be cured of by acupuncturing the right side, and vice versa" (*Plain Questions*, Chapter 5). And "diseases in the upper parts of the body can be cured of by treating the lower parts, and vice versa" (*Spiritual Pivot*, Chapter 9). The reasons are that *yin* meridians and *yang* meridians are in close relation and are the bridge to link the left and the right, as well as the upper and the lower. All these therapeutic principles embody the concept of holism.

4.1.1.7 The Wholeness in Health Maintenance

Besides treatment, TCM also values holism in health maintenance. For one thing, it emphasizes proper exercise, because insufficient exercise will lead to dysfunction of the spleen, and thus brings about systemic sickness. The spleen governs four limbs, whose exercises therefore can enhance the function of the spleen to transport and transform nutrients, which are absorbed and transformed into sufficient *qi* and blood to nourish the whole body. For another, TCM lays stress on mental tranquility. The heart is the dominator of the whole body. Only when the heart-spirit keeps tranquil, will five *zang*-organs and six *fu*-organs be in harmony. All these methods of healthcare are the reflection of the concept of holism.

In a word, the integrity of the human body itself lies in the fact that parts of the human body, composed of such substances as *qi*, blood, body fluids, are related in physical structure, coordinating and restricting in their functional activities, and mutually influential in their pathological changes.

4.1.2 The Unity of Man and Nature

The concept of holism not only refers to the integrity of the human body itself, but also the unity of the human body and nature. Man is the product of natural evolution, and has the same material property as nature. Therefore, the changes in nature have a direct or indirect effect on the functional activities of the human body, which is forced to make corresponding reactions, normal within the physiological threshold, otherwise pathological. The unity of man and nature is expressed in *The Classic of Internal Medicine* as "man correlates with heaven and earth, and corresponds with the shift of the sun and the moon." It can be expounded in two aspects: the natural and social impacts on man's physiological activities.

4.1.2.1 Natural Impact on the Human Body

The unity of man and nature is also called "correspondence between man and nature" in TCM. For one thing, human survival and reproduction totally depend on the following conditions: the physical conditions (such as space, gravity, magnetic field, temperature, air and water, etc.); the chemical conditions (such as elemental abundance, compounds, and organism); and biological conditions (biosphere and food chain). These conditions are prerequisite to normal life activities. For another, mankind is the product of the interaction of celestial *qi* and terrestrial *qi*, *yin*, and *yang*, as well as their regular movements and changes. Therefore, human beings are subject to and have to adapt to natural laws.

That life originates from nature is one important proposition for ancient Chinese philosophers. It is said in *Zhuang Zi: Zhi Bei You* that "the existence of human beings is determined by *qi*. Its accumulation ensures life, while its dispersion causes death," from which the authors of *The Classic of Internal Medicine* drew a conclusion that everything in the world including human beings was the product of nature. The same idea is stated in *Plain Questions*, Chapter 68, "man comes from *qi jiao*," where descending celestial *qi* and ascending terrestrial *qi* converge. It is *qi jiao* that causes the wane and wax of *yin* and *yang*, and produces five basic elements (wood, fire, earth, metal, water), based on which four distinct seasons are formed and human beings live. Over 2,000 years ago, authors of *The Classic of Internal Medicine* were not aware of the concept of biological evolution, and they only intuitively perceived that everything in the nature originates in a certain way. That "the interaction of celestial *qi* and terrestrial *qi* makes everything come into being" (*Plain Questions*, Chapter 2) indicates that the movements and changes of nature provide the material basis and natural conditions for everything (including human beings) to generate, develop, and change. "The world depends on the energy from the sun to go around" (*Plain Questions*, Chapter 3); "the heavens provides human beings with five kinds of energy, and the earth provides human beings with foods of five tastes (pungency, bitterness, sweetness, sourness, and saltiness)" (*Plain Questions*, Chapter 9). They all emphasize the significance of natural conditions in the life process.

Things, including life, vary with the distinct temporal and spatial conditions where they generate, grow and die. *Plain Questions*, Chapter 22 points out that the flourishing and declining of visceral *qi* occurs in different temporal and spatial dimensions. Namely, man is coherent with nature, *yin-qi* and *yang-qi* are the roots of life, and their interaction is the basis for life movements and changes.

Natural impact on the human body is reflected in several aspects, among which natural climate and geographic environment are the most obvious ones.

Living things have to adapt themselves to the seasonal variations. Spring pertains to wood, characterized by warmth; summer pertains to fire, characterized by heat; late summer pertains to earth, characterized by dampness; autumn pertains to metal, characterized by dryness; winter pertains to water, characterized by cold. Therefore, warmth in spring, heat in summer, dampness in late summer, dryness in autumn, as well as cold in winter, reveal the general law of the seasonal variations in a year. Accordingly, sprouting occurs in spring, growth in summer, transformation in late summer, reaping in autumn, and storing in winter.

Likewise, human beings change to adapt to the seasons. First, it is reflected in the changes of body fluids, e.g., "The muscular interstices open when one wears thick clothes in summer, and that is why there is sweating; the muscular interstices close when it becomes cold, and that is why dampness cannot be excreted and water is retained in the bladder to form urine or to cause retention of urine" (*Spiritual Pivot*, Chapter 36). This shows that in spring and summer, *yang-qi* is in predominance, and *qi* and blood tend to flow in the superficies, manifested as loose skin, open sweat pores and profuse sweating, etc. In autumn and winter, *yang-qi* is stored, so *qi* and blood tend to flow inside, manifested as tense skin, frequent urination, scanty sweating, etc.

Second, the pulse varies from season to season: "In spring, pulse is floating up like fish swimming under the water surface; in summer, the pulse is on the skin, more than enough; in autumn, the pulse sinks slightly under the skin like a hibernating worm entering the hole; in winter, the pulse sinks to the bone, like a hibernating worm hiding in the hole" (*Plain Questions*, Chapter 17). Pulse appears floating and strong in spring and summer, sunken and weak in autumn and winter, which are the adaptations to the alternation of four seasons through blood and *qi*.

Third, the flow of *qi* and blood in the human body also relate to the seasonal variation in the form of wind, rain, dimness, brightness, e.g., "If it is fine and sunny, the blood circulation will be smooth and the defensive *qi* will be abundant; if it is cold or cloudy, the blood circulation will be stagnated and the defensive *qi* will be sunken and hiding" (*Plain Questions*, Chapter 26).

The alternation of day and night also affects the human body, which can be expounded in terms of *yin* and *yang*. For example, "if we divide one day into four periods, dawn corresponds with spring, noon to summer, dusk to fall, and midnight to winter" (*Spiritual Pivot*, Chapter 44). Although the temperature changes in day and night are less obvious than those in the four seasons, they do show certain impacts on the human body, e.g., "*yang-qi* governs the exterior in the day time, which begins to emerge at dawn, prospers at noon, grows weak at dusk, and henceforth the sweat pore closes" (*Plain Questions*, Chapter 3).

Regional climates and geographical environments also affect the human body's physiological activities. The climate in the Yangtze River region, for example, is damp and hot, and therefore a human's muscular interstices are loose; North China is dry and cold, so the muscular interstices are dense. That is why people need some time to adapt themselves to a new place.

TCM holds that man adapts to the changes of the nature aspiringly and actively, rather than negatively and passively. Such an attitude enables them to figure out many valuable measures to improve their health and prevent diseases, for example, "to take physical activities to avoid the cold, and to live in the cool place to avoid summer-heat" (*Plain Questions*, Chapter 13); "man should live in the solid house without any cracks to evade wind and rain"

4.1 The Concept of Holism

(*Valuable Prescriptions for Emergency*[71]); "house must always be maintained clean, and in summer, it is kept open, while in winter, it is closed and kept warm" (*A New Book on Health Preservation for Old People*)[72]; "retained fluid as well as the pertinacious illness may result in new diseases; and if the ditch is well dredged and the house is kept clean, people will be away from pestilence" (*A Book on Health Preserving*)[73]. All of these are concrete measures that people take to adapt to nature.

Though seasonal climatic changes are important for living things' sprouting, growing, transforming, and reaping, they may also become adverse factors to human beings, for man's capacity to adapt to the natural environment, namely, the self-regulation function, is limited. Failing to adapt themselves to the drastic climatic changes, human beings may suffer diseases.

Seasonal changes can cause some seasonal or epidemic diseases. "Epistaxis tends to occur in spring; the disease in the chest and hypochondrium easily happens in midsummer; acute diarrhea and endogenous cold diseases often happen in late summer; wind-malaria disease is mostly seen in autumn; and in winter arthralgia syndrome often arises" (*Plain Questions*, Chapter 4). In addition, certain chronic diseases, such as arthralgia syndrome and asthma, often break out due to drastic climate changes or the sudden alternation of seasons.

The alternation of day and night also has an impact on the progression of disease to a certain extent. "As to various diseases, most of them are light at dawn and stable in the daytime, aggravate in the evening and get worse at night." That's because "at dawn, *yang-qi* of the human body begins to form and the pathogenic factors decline; during the daytime *yang-qi* grows and defeats the pathogenic factors; in the evening, *yang-qi* starts to decline and the pathogenic factors begins to generate; at night, *yang-qi* is stored into the viscera and the pathogenic factors reside alone in the body" (*Spiritual Pivot*, Chapter 44). Obviously, the conditions of disease varies with the changes of *yang-qi* in the day and night.

In addition to the seasonal and climatic factors, the geographical environment may cause some endemic diseases, too. For example, "South China, the place suitable for the growth, is abundant in *yang-qi*, low-lying in terrain, foggy and dewy. People there prefer sour and fermented food. That is why their skin is dense and red, and they are likely to suffer obstructive syndrome with muscle contracture" (*Plain Questions*, Chapter 12).

Geographically, Northwest China features high terrain, low temperature, and humidity, while Southeast China has low terrain, high temperature, and humidity. It decides that people in different regions differ in the susceptibility to different diseases, and they differ in different clinical manifestations even with the same disease, which is why doctors should use different therapeutic methods to treat the same disease in different geographical environments.

Because of such an opposite but unified relationship between man and nature, treating in accordance with season, climate, and geographical environment becomes an important principle of TCM therapeutics. Therefore, while treating based on syndrome differentiation, the relation between the external environment and the internal entirety must be taken into much consideration.

4.1.2.2 Social Impacts on the Human Body

Human beings are constituents of society, which on the one hand is affected by man, and on the other hand affects man's life.

First of all, the progress of society brings much benefit to people's health. When food and clothes become increasingly abundant for people to choose, and the inhabiting conditions become more comfortable, people are more likely to be in a healthier condition. Besides, the more people know about themselves, diseases, and the ways to stay healthy, the likelier they however, social advances may also bring about many side-effects threatening health, such as the noise produced by power-driven vehicles, the pollution of environment from industrial development, and excessive life stress. These problems, in turn, urge TCM to produce more effective measures. A case in point is that when it is found that those of rich kidney-qi are resistible to deafness caused by intense noise, TCM advocates reinforcing the kidney. Another example is that the excessive life stress can bring on various diseases like anxiety, headache, and dizziness. TCM found *qigong* and *taiji boxing* can be employed to relax both muscle and mind.

Second, peace or turmoil the society has great impacts on the human body. In a stable society, people have a regular life and strong immunity, so they are less likely to get ill and more likely to have a longer life span. In contrast, in a chaotic society where people lead an irregular life, immunity decreases, so it is easy for people to get ill and have a high mortality. World history has witnessed the physiological impacts of wars, i.e., countless people died from destitution and homelessness, irregular diet, overstrain, and pestilence.

Third, the change of an individual's social status inevitably brings about the change of his material and spiritual life, and thus affects his health indirectly. This has been taken into consideration in the diagnosis of TCM, e.g., "Before diagnosis, one must inquire of the patient of his social conditions. If the patient turns from noble to humble, though he has not been attacked by exogenous pathogenic factors, he may suffer the so-called *exhaustion of ying*. If the patient changes from rich to poor, he may suffer the so-called depletion of essence. Both diseases are due to the depression of spirit and the gradual accumulation of the stagnated energy and blood" (*Plain Questions*, Chapter 77). Therefore, the ancient Chinese claimed that to stay healthy, a person should not lay too much emphasis on wealth and rank. "When one is completely free from desires, ambitions and distracting thoughts, indifferent to fame and gain, congenital energy will maintain. When one keeps a sound mind, how can any illness occur" (*Plain Questions*, Chapter 1)?

To sum up, TCM takes the human body as an organic integrity, which is governed by the heart and centers around the five *zang*-organs. Meanwhile, it maintains that a human is inseparable from nature and society. This concept of holism runs through every field of TCM, and has become one of the basic features of the theoretical system of TCM.

4.2 Treatment Based on Syndrome Differentiation (TSD)

Treatment based on syndrome differentiation (TSD), a unique method to analyze, study, and treat diseases under the guidance of the concept of holism, is the fundamental principle of disease identification and treatment, and one of the basic features of TCM.

Syndrome differentiation is a prerequisite to treatment, while treatment is the aim of syndrome differentiation and the test of syndrome differentiation. They are inseparable in diagnosis and treatment.

To understand the concept of syndrome, a comparison has to be made between disease, syndrome, and symptom. Disease is a complete process including the specific etiology, the form of onset, pathogenesis, development, and prognosis. The typical cases of diseases are cold, dysentery, malaria, measles, asthma, and apoplexy. Symptom is the concrete clinical manifestations of diseases, like fever, cough, headache, dizziness, aching waist, and fatigue. Syndrome, different from the former two, refers to the summary of pathological changes of a disease at a certain stage in the course of its development, involving the cause (such as wind-cold, wind-heat, blood stasis, retention of phlegm, and rheum), location (the exterior, the interior, a certain *zang*-organ, a certain fu-organ, a certain meridian and, so on), the nature of a disease (such as cold, heat, etc.), as well as the relationship between pathogenic factors and vital energy (deficiency and excess, etc.). Therefore, compared with disease, syndrome is more specific and easier to be identified, and compared with symptom, it is more profound and accurate, and thus is more likely to reflect the essence of disease.

TSD, as its name implies can be divided into two stages: syndrome differentiation and treatment. The former means that by analyzing and synthesizing the clinical data of symptoms and physical signs collected through the four diagnostic methods (namely inspection, auscultation and olfaction, interrogation, and pulse taking and palpation), a doctor makes a diagnosis of syndrome based on the determination of cause, nature, and location of a disease as well as the relationship between pathogenic factors and vital energy. The latter means that a doctor decides the therapeutic methods according to the result of syndrome differentiation. These two steps are inseparable: the former is the precondition of the latter, while the latter is the aim and the test of the former.

In TCM, syndrome-differentiation-based treatment is applied more frequently than disease-differentiation-based treatment, which, as its name shows, means to decide a therapeutic method according to the diagnosis of a disease (which is effective in treating such simple diseases as ascariasis). The reason is that most diseases last long, during which the pathological changes at different stages are so varied that it is hard and inappropriate to decide on a unified therapeutic method. Such a situation requires "treating the same disease with different methods," an important aspect of TSD. The treatment of wind-warm is a good case in point. At its early stage, fever and a slight aversion to wind are the clinical manifestations of exterior wind-heat syndrome, which should be treated with drugs pungent in flavor and cool in property to relieve superficial pathogenic factors. At its middle stage, high fever, cough, shortness of breath, and dry mouth with a desire for cool drink are clinical manifestations of the exuberance of lung-heat, which should be treated by clearing lung-heat. At its late stage, the usual clinical manifestations are abatement of fever, red tongue and dry mouth, cough with scanty sputum, lassitude, and thin and weak pulse. It means that though pathogenic heat has been cleared, lung-*yin* and lung-*qi* are still in debility, and therefore the treatment should focus on clearing the remaining heat, and at the same time nourishing lung-*yin*, and reinforcing lung-*qi* as well.

TSD also involves "treating different diseases with the same method." Sometimes syndromes of different diseases are the same or similar, and therefore can be treated with the same method. For instance, both proctoptosis due to prolonged diarrhea and hysteroptosis due to improper care after confinement are caused by prolapse of gastrosplenic *qi*, so they can be treated with replenishing *qi*.

4.2.1 Specific Contents of TSD

TSD is a collective term for differentiating syndrome and treating the disease. The former involves examining the patient's condition as well as differentiating symptoms and signs, while the latter involves determining therapeutic principles and methods as well as performing the treatment.

4.2.1.1 Syndrome Differentiation

At the first stage of syndrome differentiation, to collect the clinical data of symptoms and physical signs, the doctor examines the patient's condition through the four techniques: inspection, auscultation and olfaction, interrogation, and pulse taking and palpation. It is the perceptual stage of understanding a disease, the basis to treat disease, and the prerequisite to syndrome differentiation.

- **Differentiating Symptoms and Signs**

Differentiating symptoms and signs, the rational stage of understanding a disease, means to ascertain the type of syndrome by analyzing clinical manifestations with various methods: eight-principle syndrome differentiation; disease-cause syndrome differentiation; *zang-fu* organs syndrome differentiation; *qi*-blood-body fluid syndrome differentiation; meridian-collateral syndrome differentiation; six-meridian syndrome differentiation; syndrome differentiation according to defensive phase, *qi* phase, nutrient phase and blood phase; and syndrome differentiation of *triple energizer*, etc. Whichever method is adopted, the following content and procedure are required.

Step 1: Differentiating Etiology and Pathogenesis

The name of a syndrome is ascertained according to the etiology and pathogenesis deduced from symptoms and physical signs. The process is the so-called "disease-cause syndrome differentiation." Following are some examples of syndrome concerning their disease causes: exterior syndrome due to exogenous wind-cold; toothache due to stomach-fire; diarrhea due to the deficiency of spleen-*qi*; the hyperactivity of liver-*yang*; the retention of phlegm and rheum in lungs; amenorrhea due to blood stasis; fracture due to violence; vomiting due to dyspepsia, epidemic dysentery, etc.

A disease can be ascertained according to symptoms and physical signs in terms of pathogenesis like the dysfunction of *qi* transformation, the disharmony between *yin* and *yang*, the disturbance of the normal relationship between *qi* and blood, and the disorder of functions of *zang-fu* organs, etc.

Step 2: Differentiating the Location of a Disease

It means to ascertain the location where disease occurs. Different pathogenic factors may attack different body parts and end up with varied syndromes. For instance, it is said in *Plain Questions*, Chapter 5 that "the climatic pathogens often attack the human body from the exterior first, and then to the interior, and finally to the five *zang*-organs. Taking food or drink of improper temperature may cause disease of stomach and intestine. Retained pathogenic dampness will impair skin, muscle, tendon and meridians." And it is also said in *Plain Questions*, Chapter 29 that "when asthenia-pathogenic wind invades the human body, it will affect *yang* meridians first, and then six *fu*-organs, which will cause fever, insomnia and dyspnea; improper diet or irregular life will do harm to *yin* meridians and then five *zang*-organs, which will cause distention of abdomen, lienteric diarrhea, and even dysentery." "Pathogenic wind always attacks the upper parts of the body, while pathogenic dampness mostly affects the lower parts." The precise judgment of the location of disease enables us to learn the cause and transmission of a disease and thus helps us to improve our treatment.

Step 3: Differentiating the Nature of a Disease

The nature of a disease refers to the state of pathogenic factors and that of vital energy. In TCM, *yin-yang* is the general guiding principle; cold and heat, as well as deficiency and excess are the natures to be differentiated.

Yin-yang is the general guiding principle in that pathogenic factors are either *yin* or *yang* in nature, so does vital energy. Excess syndrome and heat syndrome pertain to *yang*, while deficiency syndrome and cold syndrome to *yin*. Cold and heat syndromes are the results of the changes between *yin* and *yang*, and deficiency and excess syndromes are the manifestations of the struggle between vital energy (*yin*) and pathogenic factors (*yang*). *Plain Questions*, Chapter 5 holds that an experienced physician always starts a diagnosis with distinguishing the *yin* syndrome and *yang* syndrome through observing the complexion and palpating the pulse.

Cold syndrome can be divided into two types: excess-cold syndrome caused by the exuberance of pathogenic cold, and deficiency-cold syndrome caused by the declination of *yang-qi* and the depletion of vital energy. Heat syndrome can also be divided into excessive-heat syndrome due to the exuberance of pathogenic heat, and deficiency-heat syndrome due to the insufficiency of *yin*-fluid and the weakness of vital energy.

Only by understanding the nature of a disease, can we decide appropriate therapeutic principles: "treating cold syndrome with warm therapy and heat syndrome with cold therapy"; "treating deficiency syndrome with supplementation therapy and excess syndrome with purgation therapy"; "treating *yang* disease from *yin* aspect and *yin* disease from *yang* aspect," etc. These principles effectively guide the composition of prescriptions and the selection of herbs.

- **Differentiating the State of a Disease**

Differentiating the state of a disease is a general consideration of a disease in a quantitative sense. Due to the limitation of ancient metric means, physicians could only make a rough judgment of a disease by the four methods of examination (namely inspection, auscultation and olfaction, interrogation, and pulse taking and palpation); make a vague description about the extent of pathological changes (such as shallow and deep, light and severe, acute and chronic); and then determine the therapeutic principle, prescription, and herb. At that time, numbers could be directly used to describe the amount of pathogenic factors or vital energy, for example, "no more herbs with great toxicity should be applied when pathogenic factors are removed by 60%; those with small toxicity should be ceased when pathogenic factors are removed by 70%; common herbs are not necessary when pathogenic factors are removed by 80%; herbs without any toxicity should be ceased when pathogenic factors are removed by 90%" (*Plain Questions*, Chapter 70). The percentages like 60%, 70%, 80%, and 90% refer to the rough ratio of pathogenic factors. The fuzziness lays the foundation for the study of TCM in a mathematical way, that is, to establish the mathematic model for differentiating and diagnosing with the aid of a computer.

- **Differentiating the Developmental Tendency of a Disease**

Differentiating the tendency of disease development means to identify the developmental trend and evolutionary direction of a disease. It involves the following three aspects: the developmental speed, trend, and the dynamism of a disease.

As far as the developmental speed is concerned, under normal circumstances, exogenous diseases and *yang* syndrome develop quickly, while the disease due to internal injury and *yin* syndrome have to experience a prolonged course. Such laws decide that urgent remedies should be made.

The developmental trend of a disease refers to the course or phase with varied syndromes. For example, exogenous diseases, according to *The Classic of Internal Medicine*, experience six phases. In terms of Six Meridians they are *Taiyang*, *Yangming*, *Shaoyang*, *Taiyin*, *Shaoyin*, and *Jueyin* meridians. Epidemic febrile diseases and damp-heat diseases experience defensive phase, *qi* phase, nutrient phase, and blood phase, as well as *triple energizer*. The transmission of internal-injury diseases, according to *The Classic of Internal Medicine*, is carried out in the form of generating, restricting, subjugating, and reverse restricting among Five Elements. For these developmental trends, we should take the initiative to control the disease by cutting off potential development and preventing deterioration. For example, one important TCM therapeutic principle is "to strengthen the function of non-infected viscera first" (*Treatise on Pestilence*). Specifically, "measures must be taken to strengthen the function of the spleen in the treatment of liver disease, or to keep the spleen off pathogenic factors," for "the pathological factors of the liver are likely to transmit to the spleen" (*Synopsis of Golden Chamber*, Chapter 1).

The dynamism of a disease and syndrome refers to such alterations of pathogenesis as ascending, descending, going out, and coming in. We choose herbal drugs with the natures of lifting, lowering, floating, and sinking correspondingly.

- **Differentiating Superficiality and Origin**

Superficiality and origin are terms peculiar to TCM. They refer to contradictory unities, i.e., primary and secondary, fundamental and incidental, mild and severe, and greater and less urgency of the processes of physiology, pathology, and treatment. In the development of a disease, an origin is fundamental, determining the nature and developmental trend, while superficiality is secondary, reflecting the development speed in a certain sense. Based on the differentiation of superficiality and origin, clinical procedures are determined: "treating the incidental under urgent situation, and treating the fundamental under milder situation," because the incidental symptom is too acute to be overlooked, otherwise it may affect or even turn to the principal aspect of the contradiction following the law of "transformation of superficiality and origin." The mastery of the method of differentiating superficiality and origin enables us to treat complicated cases accurately in the order of seriousness and urgency.

- **Differentiating the Syndrome of a Disease**

It refers to the diagnostic process and result in which diseases and syndromes are ascertained and specifically named. According to *Plain Questions*, Chapter 80, the complete procedure can be described in detail as: identifying the cause and location of a disease based on the systemic checkup; observing its tendency as well as its superficiality and origin; ascertaining its pathogenesis consistent with symptoms and physical signs; and finally naming a disease and syndrome correctly. That is, the result of diagnosis should fully reflect the cause, location, and pathogenesis of a disease. For example, the diagnosis of dysentery is determined by its location (intestine), cause (cold dysentery, heat dysentery, damp-heat dysentery, or epidemic dysentery), and its pathogenesis differentiation (like *qi* stagnation dysentery, blood stasis dysentery, and anorectic dysentery).

The above rational understandings are continuous steps of dialectical thinking in TCM. They reflect the nature and the intrinsic relation of a disease from different perspectives.

4.2.1.2　　Treatment

To treat a disease is to decide the corresponding therapeutic principles and methods according to the result of syndrome differentiation.

- **Determining Specific Therapeutic Principles**

The general therapeutic principles are therapeutic guidelines for any treatment: "to focus on the principal cause of disease"; "to strengthen vital energy to eliminate pathogenic factors"; "to regulate *yin* and *yang*"; "to select the proper therapy according to individuality, time and geographical environment," etc. Under the guidance of the general therapeutic principles, specific therapeutic principles should be determined according to the specific name of a specific disease and the specific pattern of syndrome. For example, the external excess syndrome can be specifically divided into the exterior wind-cold syndrome and the exterior wind-heat syndrome. Guided by the general principle, "to eliminate pathogenic factors by strengthening vital energy," their respective therapeutic principles are either relieving superficial pathogenic factors with drugs pungent in flavor and warm in property, or relieving superficial pathogenic factors with drugs pungent in flavor and cool in property.

- **Deciding the Therapeutic Means and Prescriptions**

Once therapeutic principles are determined, the therapeutic means and prescriptions will be decided accordingly. Therapeutic means include both drug and nondrug therapies. The former can be used internally or externally, while the latter covers various approaches, such as acupuncture, moxibustion, massage, *qigong*, etc. To compose prescriptions is to write out the concrete ways of treatment according to the selected therapeutic means. For instance, for drug therapy, it includes the formula, name, and dosage of every ingredient, the method of processing medicinal materials, the time of taking medicine, and the daily dosage,

4.2 Treatment Based on Syndrome Differentiation (TSD)

etc; for nondrug therapy, it involves the name of the approach, the location of treatment, manipulation techniques, the degree and duration. Each therapy has its own characteristics.

- **Carrying out Treatment**

It refers to the process of carrying out the therapy according to the prescription, e.g., decocting Chinese medicinal herbs, applying the medicine externally, fumigating, selecting acupoints, practicing acupuncture manipulations, massaging a certain part of the body, or doing *qigong*.

A complete process of diagnosis and treatment includes examination, syndrome differentiation, and treatment. Generally speaking, a disease is hard to be recognized thoroughly and exactly at one time, and the doctor should constantly adjust the methods according to the feedback in treatment. That is why TCM attaches much importance to inquiring into the patient's response to the last treatment and emphasizes the fact that the curative effect is the standard to test the quality of syndrome differentiation. Only in this way can the cognitive process of TSD gradually reflect the essence of a disease, and can the ability to recognize and treat the disease be constantly improved.

4.2.2 Relationship between Syndrome Differentiation and Treatment

Syndrome differentiation and treatment are the two most important elements in the application of the theory, principle, prescription, and herb of TCM, and they are interrelated and inseparable in the diagnosis and treatment of a disease. For one thing, syndrome differentiation is the prerequisite to treatment. Only with correct syndrome differentiation can proper therapeutic principles and methods be determined, and the remarkable therapeutic effect be achieved. For another, treatment is the aim of syndrome differentiation, and its effect is the standard to check the correctness of syndrome differentiation and treatment. Therefore, TSD embodies the organic combination of theory and practice.

4.2.3 The Principles of TSD

Although it is hard to differentiate complex and changeable syndromes, it doesn't mean that syndrome cannot be understood. As long as certain principles are guided, accurate syndrome differentiation and the right treatment can be accomplished. The principles of TSD are stated as follows.

4.2.3.1 Guided by Holism, Based on Systematic Theories

The guideline of TSD is the view of holism of TCM, namely the human body is an organic integrity. United with nature, the human body is influenced by the natural conditions and therefore has to adapt to the natural law, such as the unceasing operation of celestial bodies, the shift of the sun and moon, the alteration between winter and summer, as well as the wane and wax of *yin* and *yang*. Diseases vary with the changes of the natural and social environments, the state of the human body, and the medical conditions. Based on such a holism, the essence of diseases can be identified and the specific treatment can be determined. Moreover, systematic TCM theories are the basis of TSD. To be specific, the location of a disease is ascertained according to the physiological structure; the nature of a disease is ascertained based on the physiological dysfunction and the nature of pathogenic factors; the developmental trend of a disease and the prognosis are deduced by analyzing the pathology and the state of vital energy; and then the diagnostic result is obtained through syndrome differentiation. Based on them, therapeutic principles, specific means, and prescriptions are decided.

4.2.3.2　Following the Law of Syndrome

To grasp the law of disease evolution and to differentiate the characteristics of syndromes more accurately, a doctor must understand the law of syndrome in a comprehensive way.

- **The Variability of Syndrome**

Syndrome, an integral concept of pathology, is a pathological summary of a disease at a certain stage of development, involving the cause, location, and nature of a disease as well as the relationship between pathogenic factors and vital energy. It is a dynamic reflection of the holistic effect of pathogenic factors on the human body. Etiologically, syndromes may vary with environmental changes (both natural and social), emotional disturbance, and the rhythm of daily routines; pathogenically, the changes of syndromes may be caused by the mutual-influence of local and whole pathological changes; pathologically, syndromes may change involving the changes of structure and function, such as the morphological change of some parts of the human body or an abnormal change of physical functions.

The variability of syndrome can be fully reflected in the transmission and transformation of diseases of Six Meridians as well as their changes from simplicity to complexity. Diseases of Six Meridians, namely, *Taiyang* disease, *Yangming* disease, *Shaoyang* disease, *Taiyin* disease, *Shaoyin* disease, and *Jueyin* disease, are the six stages of pathological changes on the basis of the integrity of syndrome. Each meridian not only relates to a certain organ and its function, but also connects with other meridians. Therefore, diseases of Six Meridians are both independent and closely related to each other. Each of them may develop longitudinally along its course and manifest different syndromes. It is called "the same disease with different syndromes," and the opposite case is called "the different diseases with the same syndrome."

- **The Stability of Syndrome**

Besides variability, stability is also the law of syndrome. Syndrome, the reflection of a disease at a certain stage, is in a relatively stable state, which is the foundation of syndrome differentiation. Each syndrome pattern is the specific manifestation of the stability of syndrome.

4.2.3.3　Combining Syndrome Differentiation and Disease Differentiation

TSD, a principle of diagnosis and treatment unique to TCM, guides practitioners to understand the relationship between disease and syndrome dialectically. Since a disease may manifest itself as various syndromes and different diseases may have the same syndrome, both disease differentiation and syndrome differentiation should be taken into consideration in the understanding and treatment of diseases.

Disease differentiation enables us to have a macroscopic understanding of a disease, so that we can make correct syndrome differentiation, compose appropriate prescriptions, and choose proper herbs. A good case in point is the differentiation and treatment of Behcet's disease, whose syndromes may be the erosion of the throat, anus, and genitalia. Without correct disease differentiation, the erosion of genitalia may be taken for gynecologic, surgical, and anorectal diseases; likewise, the erosion of the throat may be misunderstood as a laryngological diseases, which may lead to ineffective treatment, or even deterioration.

However, correct disease differentiation alone cannot guarantee the treatment. For example, without syndrome differentiation, mania cannot be treated effectively only by disease differentiation, for no proper means can be determined without an understanding of the etiological, pathogenic, and pathological factors of the disease in its development. Mania in Chinese is "癫狂"; the name is determined mostly based on the main features of the disease. The manifestations of "癫" are depression, expressionlessness, inclination for quietness, self-muttering, fantasizing and hallucinating, caprice in crying and laughing, paraphasia, loss of appetite, unawareness of filth and cleanness, etc. Different from "癫," "狂." is marked by violent attacks of fury, ravings, even fierceness, ascending a height to sing, walking naked, polyphagia, anorexia, visual and auditory delusion, audaciousness and restlessness, red tongue with yellow and greasy coating, taut, slippery and rapid pulse or deep, tense and replete pulse, etc. Without a correct differentiation of syndromes, a doctor cannot tell whether the disease was caused by anxiety and melancholy, or the impairment of the heart and spleen, or stasis of phlegm-*qi* and heart confused by phlegm, or it is caused by the excess of *seven emotions*, fire-transmission from the disorder of *five emotions*, the heart confused by phlegm, or pathogen in the heart due to excessive heat.

Disease and syndrome are not equal but intrinsically interrelated. Though they are not in the relationship of universality and individuality, nor cause and result, they are related as process and stage, and whole and local. Therefore, both of their differentiations should be taken seriously in diagnosis and treatment. The style of the book *Treatise on Exogenous Febrile Disease and Miscellaneous Disease* by Zhang Zhongjing presents us a good model. Every section of the book is named after "Treatment of XX Disease Firstly Based on Disease Differentiation and then on Syndrome Differentiation," which informs learners of the order of diagnosis and treatment. Ye Gui, one founder of the School of Seasonal Febrile Disease in the Qing dynasty, also pointed out that disease differentiation had the guiding significance for syndrome differentiation, for a disease might display various syndromes, which are changeable in the development of the disease. Syndrome differentiation under the guidance of disease differentiation enables us to grasp the overall situation, to clarify gradations, to avoid mistakes, and thus to improve diagnosis and treatment. Therefore, disease differentiation and syndrome differentiation form a dialectical unity in diagnosis.

4.2.3.4 Treatment on Principles with Necessary Adaptation

For one thing, in treatment, the general therapeutic principles such as "focusing on the principal cause of disease" are to be abided by. The reason is that despite the complexity of structure and function of the human body and the consequent variability of diseases, the general causes of diseases are similar and can be generalized into the exuberance of pathogenic factors and the declination of vital energy, or the imbalance between *yin* and *yang*. The general therapeutic principles, however, are not rigid, for in the view of holism, different patterns of syndrome result from the different constitution and pathogenic factors, time variation, and geographical and social environments. Therefore, "selecting the proper therapy according to individuality, time and geographical environment" becomes another general principle we should follow.

For another, physicians should make necessary adaptations to syndromes sometimes, while following the general principles. Since a disease constantly changes, and may display various syndromes in its development. And causes for the syndromes may also be varied: the wane and wax of *yin* and *yang*; or the exuberance and declination of pathogenic factors and vital energy. Syndrome differentiation and adaptation should be carried out until the patient is fully recovered. The variability of syndrome requires adaptive therapeutic strategies, such as "treating the same disease with the same method," "treating different diseases with different methods," "treating the same disease with different methods," and "treating different diseases with the same method."

One important thing should be born in mind: the general therapeutic principles are a must for any medical physician in specific therapies, a warming therapy or a cooling therapy, a supplementing therapy or a purging therapy. However the insistence on general principles does not deny the adaptability and adaptability of syndromes. Abiding by principle and adaptability form a dialectical unity in pathogenesis. Only when they are organically combined, can therapeutic methods be more proper, prescriptions more accurate, and curative effects more notable.

4.2.4 Superiority of TSD

The superiority of TSD is shown in the following two aspects.

For one thing, TSD contains some peculiar and advanced methods like the "black box method" (a method of exploring the internal structure and mechanism by observing the relation between the external input information and output information), and the "feedback adjustment method" (a method of adjusting the system by responding to the perturbation in the same direction as the perturbation or the opposite direction), which are the embryos of the modern interdisciplinary subject.

For another, TSD has the characteristic of fuzziness, which will make the application of fuzzy mathematics and computers in TCM possible, and therefore promote the academic modernization of TCM.

CHAPTER 5

Philosophical Foundation of TCM

Objectives & Requirements
1. Philosophical foundation of TCM.
2. Formation, development, essential contents, and application of the theory of primordial *qi*.
3. Formation, development, essential contents, and application of *yin-yang* theory.
4. Formation, development, essential contents, and application of the theory of Five-Elements.
5. Interrelationships among theories of primordial *qi*, *yin-yang* and Five Elements.

Key Concepts
1. The philosophical doctrines of primordial *qi*, *yin-yang*, and Five Elements not only deeply influence TCM but also become its leading philosophical methods.
2. The doctrine of primordial *qi* (also called monism of *qi*) holds that as the origin of everything, *qi* is in constant motion, and the law of the motion and change of *qi* is called "Tao." The theory of primordial *qi* runs through such aspects of TCM as physiology, pathology, diagnosis, and treatment.
3. *Yin-yang* is the summary of the opposing sides of some interrelated things and phenomena in nature. The theory involves *yin-yang* interaction, opposition, interdependence, wane-wax, and mutual-transformation. It is used to explain the histological structure, physiological functions, and pathological changes of the human body and guide clinical diagnosis and treatment effectively.
4. The theory of Five Elements classifies things into five categories (wood, fire, earth, metal, and water) according to their properties. The basic contents of the theory can be generalized into interpromotion, interrestraint, overrestraint, and counterrestraint. The theory of Five Elements can be applied to expound TCM theory and to guide clinical treatment.
5. The theories of primordial *qi*, *yin-yang*, and Five Elements have promoted the establishment and development of TCM's theoretical system and are of great value in clinical practice. As a natural view, the theory of primordial *qi* lays the theoretical fundament for TCM; as methodology, the theories of *yin-yang* and Five Elements establish the basic framework for TCM's theoretical system.

Philosophically TCM originated from the ancient doctrines of primordial *qi*, *yin-yang*, and Five Elements. The doctrine of primordial *qi*, monism of the origin of the world, holds that everything in the world is made up of *qi*, whose constant movement and change cause the corresponding motion and change of the cosmos. The doctrine of *yin-yang*, dualism of the origin of the world, holds that everything in the world can be divided into the aspects of *yin* and *yang* that are opposite but interdependent; and the things' nature can also be classified into *yin* and *yang*, and then named as *yin* or *yang* to show their dominance in the proportion. The dominance is changeable with the wane and wax between *yin* and *yang*, and can turn to the opposite in the *yin-yang* transformation. The doctrine of Five Elements, the pluralism of the origin of the world, maintains that the cosmos is composed of wood, fire, earth, metal, and water; they are interpromoting and interrestraining, making the universe in a dynamic balance. These three philosophical doctrines not only deeply influence TCM but also become the leading philosophical methods in TCM, penetrating all the areas of TCM.

5.1 The Theory of Primordial Qi

The theory of primordial qi is the theoretical guideline for ancient philosophers to understand the origin of the universe. Early in *A Book of Changes*,[74] qi was introduced as a philosophical notion. Since then, qi had been studied thoroughly. The theory of primordial qi was preliminarily formed as a natural view in the pre-Qin dynasty. It has had a profound influence on the formation of TCM's theoretical system and becomes one of the most important concepts and contents of TCM.

5.1.1 The Formation and Development of the Theory of Primordial Qi

Qi appeared as a philosophical notion in the literatures of the pre-Qin dynasty, such as *On Leud States*,[75] which explained the earthquake in the 8th century B.C. as "the disorder of celestial qi and terrestrial qi." Yi He, a famous physician of the Qin dynasty, pointed out that every visible thing was generated from six kinds of changeable and invisible qi, i.e., *yin*, *yang*, wind, rain, darkness, and brightness. Likewise, Zhuang Zhou, a philosopher in the middle of the Warring States Period, also maintained that the visible substances originated from the changes of invisible qi. In addition, he attributed the life process to the accumulation and dispersion of qi (*Chuang-tzu*).[76]

After Zhuang Zhou, the notion of Qi was further understood. *He Guan Zi*[77] called it "primordial qi," namely, qi is the origin of the universe. Thereafter, this viewpoint was adequately affirmed by philosophers of the Han dynasty, Liu Xin, Wang Chong, and He Xiu. After the Qin and Han dynasties, the theory was further developed. Many philosophers of the Eastern and Western Han dynasties agreed that with qi as an intermediary, the same kind of things can interact with each other. Liu Zongyuan, a philosopher of the Tang dynasty, advanced the idea that "nothing but primordial qi exists before the formation of the cosmos."

In the Song dynasty, owing to the endeavors of such philosophers as Zhang Zai, the theory of primordial qi was developed into a natural materialism. Zhang Zai, a synthesizer of various thoughts of qi monism, named the process of qi change as Tao, where the qi's dispersing and invisible pristine condition is *Taixu* (nothingness), and its accumulating and visible state form everything. These viewpoints permeate such aspects as the relationships of qi and shape, qi and nature, qi and spirit, and qi and law.

In the late Ming dynasty and the early Qing dynasty, the development of the theory was attributed to such philosophers as Wang Fuzhi who emphasized that everything including "mind," "character," and other psychological and personal characteristics are derivatives of qi.

5.1.2 The Basic Contents of the Theory of Primordial Qi

The theory of primordial qi reflects an ancient people's basic understanding of nature including human life and the morbidity process.

5.1.2.1 Qi is the Origin of the World

The ancient Chinese philosophers held that primordial qi was the most essential substance to constitute the universe. The boundless universe is filled with qi, whose constant motion creates the hosts of heaven, the seasonal changes, and spectacular scenes of nature. It is not exaggerating to say that primordial qi and its motion are the origin of the generation and variation of all things in the natural world: birds in the sky, animals on the land, rare jewels, varied plants, and even intelligent human beings.

Ancient Chinese philosophers classified natural substances into "visible substances" and "invisible substances" (or "nothingness"). Invisible Qi accumulates and forms various visible things. Therefore invisible and visible objects are the same in nature, though different in the state.

5.1.2.2 Qi Is in Constant Motion

According to the theory of primordial qi, qi is not static but in constant motion, which results in the unceasing emergence of new things, constant growing from young to old, the gradual declining from strong to weak, and finally to death. *Plain Questions* states that where there is qi, there is its motion; where there is the motion of qi, there are observable objects, who are growing with the nourishment of qi and withering with its decline.

The motion and change of qi follows a certain law, which is called "Tao" by the ancient philosophers. Lao-tzu, the founder of Taoism in the Spring and Autumn Period, expounded that "man follows the principle of the earth, the earth follows that of the heaven, the heaven follows that of Tao, and Tao follows that of nature"(*Lao-tzu*, Chapter 25). Therefore it is Tao, the law of qi's movement, that regulates the states of everything, its motion and variation. *Lao-tzu*, pointed out that "one produces two, two produces three, and three produces everything in the world"; "one" is the primordial qi that gives birth to *yin-qi* and *yang-qi* through its motion and change, and then the motion of *yin-qi* and *yang-qi* produces many things, which further create all the things in the world.

The movement of qi, also called "qi activity," has various styles, such as accumulating and dispersing, ascending and descending, coming in and going out.

Accumulating and dispersing are the most essential moving styles of qi. The accumulation of qi brings on the birth of everything, while its dispersion leads to death. The complete process is that things grow with the accumulation of qi, develop to a certain extent, then disintegrate and die due to the dispersion of qi, and finally turn back to invisible qi, whose reaggregation generates another new thing in its constant movement. Like inanimate things, all living things of complicated structure and function, experience the same process.

Other moving styles of qi are ascending, descending, coming in, and going out. *Plain Questions*, Chapter 68 holds that all the things in the universe originate from qi, and their variations result from the upward, downward, inward, and outward movements of qi. Without ascending terrestrial qi, there is no descending celestial qi. The descending activity of celestial qi that produces all things on earth and ascending activity of terrestrial qi that transforms into celestial qi lead to the endless movement of all the things in the natural world.

5.1.2.3 Qi Is the Intermediary of the Natural Interaction

Ancient Chinese philosophers categorized things in terms of their natures. Things of the same or different natures interact with each other. The cases are the resonance caused by a musical instrument, an attraction between magnet and iron, fire from a concave bronze mirror in the sunlight, sea tides from the gravitational attraction of the moon and the sun, and human physiological and pathological changes affected by the variations of the sun and the moon, day and night, as well as season and climate.

Ubiquitous qi is the intermediary of various natural interactions, for it can permeate observable objects and constantly exchange with the component qi, accumulating, dispersing, ascending, descending, coming in, and going out. Besides, no matter how distant two visible objects are, with qi, interaction is possible. For example, sea tides are the response of the sea to the changes of the sun and the moon; even the crane screaming at midnight and the cock crowing at dawn all result from their reactions to light and sound produced by the movement of qi. The authors of The Classic of Internal Medicine also pointed out that qi produced human beings, who correlated to heaven and the earth, and corresponded with the shift of the sun and the moon through qi.

5.1.2.4 Life Consists in the Movement of Qi

Ancient Chinese viewed that life activities were the result of the constant and regular movement of qi. Qi-transformation is the essential cause for the production and existence of life.

Qi-transformation means changes caused by the movement of qi, which generally refers to all types of movements and changes, including qi transforming into the body, the body transforming into other bodies, the body transforming into qi, etc. In such a way qi propels the development and change of the cosmos. Invisible qi accumulating into visible objects is the process of the transformation of qi into the body, while visible objects dispersing into qi is the process of the transformation of the body into qi. Specific to the human body, birth and death also depend on the accumulating and dispersing activities of qi. The process of one body transforming into another body means that visible objects intertransform by the propelling and stimulating functions of qi. For example, through qi, body fluids can be transformed into blood, urine, or sweat; through qi, food can be changed into nutrients that human metabolism needs. All these processes are always accompanied by the accumulation, transformation, or release of energy. Thus, the process of qi-transformation is the conversion process of material and energy, which generalizes all kinds of metabolic activities.

5.1.3 The Application of the Theory of Primordial Qi in TCM

TCM inherits the philosophic theory of primordial qi and develops it into a unique medical theory. It puts forward the idea of qi, explores the law of qi activity in human physiological and pathological courses, and investigates the therapeutic methods to regulate qi in the whole body.

5.1.3.1 Explanation of Man's Production and Physiological Activity

Man originates from the motion and the variation of qi, following the law of nature. Different from other organisms produced by qi, man is composed of natural, social, and mental attributes, and therefore he is not only the unity of the body and life, but also the unity of the body and mind; he cannot only understand the nature but also dynamically reform the world. In this sense, man is the most advanced organism in the natural world. Just as Hsun Tzu interpreted, "water and fire have no life though they have qi; grass and tree have no perception though they have life; and birds and beasts have no morality though they have perception. A human being has qi, life, perception, and morality, and therefore is the most privileged."

A man's body comes from the accumulation of qi; a man's normal life activities are nourished by food and fresh air; and man's metabolism is the manifestation of qi-transformation. A man's perception, thought, emotion, and other psychological activities are also generated from the movement of qi. Plain Questions, Chapter 5 believed that "five zang-organs dominate five kinds of visceral qi to produce five types of emotions: joy, anger, grief, worry, and fear." Liu Wansu and Zhang Jiebin, the outstanding ancient Chinese physicians, all emphasized that "spirit is generated by qi" and spirit was the product of the motion of the material.

5.1.3.2 Explanation of the Cause, Onset and Pathology of Diseases

Besides mobility of the life process, the notion of qi can also be used to interpret the cause of disease and pathogenesis. First, pathogenic factors are called "evil qi," including such abnormal climatic factors as wind, cold, summer-heat, dampness, dryness and heat, and pestilence. Just as Wu Youke (a famous physician in the late Ming dynasty) said, these pathogenic factors were imperceptible but objective. Each of them may cause diseases. These understandings about the cause of disease are the embryonic form of modern microbial etiology. Second, "healthy qi" refers to the disease-resistant substance, structure and function of the human body, such as nutrient qi and defensive qi, as well as the normal physiological function of viscera. Third, the struggle between evil qi and healthy qi is the basic mechanism of the occurrence and the development of diseases; the change of asthenia and excess caused by the struggle is one of the basic pathological changes.

The state and the functional condition of qi affect various physiological phenomena or pathological processes. When qi is abundant and works well, a man will stay healthy, with sound functional activities of tissues and organs, normal body temperature, and strong disease resistibility. Conversely, when qi is deficient and does not work well, a man will get ill and cannot recover easily, with unsound functional activities of the whole body or partial organs, abnormal body temperature, and less disease resistibility. In this case, only by regulating qi, can one recover.

5.1.3.3 Guiding Clinical Diagnosis and Treatment

Different pathogenic factors, when struggling with vital energy, may cause different diseases, with different syndromes, symptoms, and physical signs. The disorder of qi activity brings about abnormal physiological manifestations such as chill, fever, pain, distress, flatulency and numbness, no appetite, and abnormal conditions of tongue and pulse. To make a diagnosis is to analyze pathological changes and judge the disease cause, pathogenesis, and syndrome pattern according to various symptoms and physical signs. To carry out a treatment is to take corresponding measures to eliminate pathogenic factors, restore vital energy, and promote rehabilitation of patients based on the diagnosis. Basic therapeutic methods can be briefly summarized as eliminating pathogenic factors, supporting vital energy, and regulating qi activity.

5.1.3.4 Guiding Health Maintenance

Medical prevention, based on scientific investigations into human physiology and pathology, is more important than diagnosis and treatment to some extent. The theory of primordial qi also accounts for the integrity of the human body and becomes one philosophical foundation of TCM's holism. As the most essential substance of the human body, qi flows continuously inside the body and accumulates to form visible organs. Therefore, in health maintenance, it is important to keep qi unobstructed, which is achieved by residing stably, keeping a balance between activity and rest, regulating diet and emotions, and exercising regularly.

5.2 The Theory of *Yin-yang*

The theory of *yin-yang* is one ancient philosophical theory in China. It studies the law of motion, occurrence, development, and variation in the cosmos.

The theory of *yin-yang* is a dialectics based on the ancient materialism. It holds that as a material integrity, the world is the unity of the opposing *yin* and *yang*, and *yin-yang* interaction promotes the occurrence and the development of things.

The philosophical doctrine of *yin-yang* permeates the medical field, combines with the TCM theories, and forms peculiar TCM's *yin-yang* view, guiding the medical cognition and practice for centuries.

5.2.1 The Origin and Formation of the *Yin-yang* Theory

The notions of *yin* and *yang* date back to the Shang dynasty. The oracle bone script contains such phrases as "dark moon" and "light sun," which express the naive thought of *yin* and *yang*. The primary connotations of *yin* and *yang* were rather simple, only referring to the location of things relevant to the sun. Facing the sun is called *yang*, otherwise it is *yin*. Since then the notions have been widely applied in daily life, for example, to judge the features of a piece of land or the direction of a current.

The symbols for *yin* and *yang*, "- -" and "—", first appeared in *A Book of Changes*. They are the divinatory symbols to form hexagram statements. In the Zhou dynasty, the compound word *yin-yang* was used frequently in daily life, poetry, and philosophy. *On Leud States* recorded that Bo Yangfu, a philosopher in the 8th century B.C., interpreted earthquake as the disharmonious movement of *yin* and *yang*, two opposing powers in the earth. The correlated movement and changes of *yin* and *yang* were named as "Tao" by *Yi Zhuan*, a reference book on *A Book of Changes*. Thereafter, *yin-yang* was universally applied to understanding and reforming nature.

Thanks to *yin-yang* experts such as Zou Yan and Zou Shi, the Warring States Period saw the establishment of the independent and systematic *yin-yang* theory. Since then, it has promoted the development of astronomy, calendar, meteorology, and agriculture (*A Record of Art and Culture, History of the Han Dynasty*).[78]

After the Eastern and Western Han dynasties, the theory of *yin-yang* developed rapidly. The following philosophers in the Song dynasty are the synthesizer of the theory. In *Taiji Diagram*,[79] Zhou Dunyi explained the relationship between *Taiji* (*qi*), *yin-yang* and Five Elements: the universe developed from Wuji (a state of Nothingness) to *Taiji*, the motion of *Taiji* generated *yin* and *yang*, then the variation of *yin* and *yang* produced Five Elements, and finally *yin-yang* and Five Elements generated everything in the world. Zhang Zai believed that every object (or phenomenon) could be divided into *yin* and *yang* aspects, which furthered the understanding of the contradictory unity relationship between *yin* and *yang*. Wang Tingxiang in the Ming dynasty proposed the idea of "dividing one into two, and combining two into one," namely there are two inseparable poles of *yin* and *yang* in the united primordial *qi*.

In the medical field, the *yin-yang* view was also developed. The idea that *yin* and *yang* were two parts of one was clearly expressed by Yang Shangshan, a famous physician of the Sui and Tang dynasties; and the systemic explanation of TCM's *Yin-yang* theory was presented by Zhang Jiebin, the outstanding physician in the Ming dynasty.

Under the guideline of *yin-yang* theory, physicians in the Spring and Autumn Period and the Warring States Period solved many medical problems. Yi He, an outstanding physician of the Qin, attributed the causes of diseases to "six kinds of *qi*" (i.e., cold, heat, wind, rain, gloominess, and drought): excess cold caused cold diseases; excess heat caused heat diseases; excess wind brought on head diseases; excess rain caused gastrointestinal diseases; prolonged gloomy days led to depression; and prolonged drought resulted in irritability. Such a viewpoint was similar to that of *The Classic of Internal Medicine*: various diseases resulted from exogenous pathogenic factors, such as cold, summer-heat, wind, rain, wetness, and dryness.

The philosophical theory of *yin-yang* opposition and unity makes a great contribution to the observation of human physiology, etiology, onset of disease, pathogenesis, syndrome, diagnosis, treatment, health maintenance, and disease prevention. With the development of TCM and the corresponding improvement of philosophical *yin-yang* theory itself, it has become a solid and an indispensable theoretical foundation of TCM.

5.2.2 The Basic Concept of *Yin-yang*

Ancient Chinese found that all objects and phenomena have two opposing aspects and termed them as *yin* and *yang*. *Yin-yang*, an abstract notion, was formed based on the common and essential attribute of concrete objects and phenomena. It neither refers to any concrete object and phenomenon, nor is any entity itself, just as *Spiritual Pivot*, Chapter 41 states, "*Yin* and *yang* are in names but not in shapes."

5.2.2.1 Conditions Categorizing *Yin* and *Yang*

The categorization of objects (or phenomena) in terms of *yin* and *yang* is not arbitrary but conditional. One condition is the correlation of objects (or phenomena), and the other is the opposition in the attribute of objects (or phenomena).

The so-called correlation refers to the interrelationship between two objects (or phenomena) or two aspects of any one object (or phenomenon). They are opposite but unified into a whole. Without such a relation, they cannot be categorized as *yin* and *yang*. For example, as for male and female, male pertains to *yang* and female to *yin*; as to the external part and internal part of one object, the external pertains to *yang* and the internal to *yin*. It is improper to distinguish between *yin* and *yang* in such pairs as male and the external, male and the internal, female and the external, as well as female and the internal, for they lack intrinsic correlation.

The so-called opposing attributes of two objects (or phenomena) refer to their opposition in quality. For instance, fire and water, and the upper and the lower are two pairs not only correlated, but also opposite in quality, and therefore they can be called *yin* and *yang*. For fire and water, fire pertains to *yang* and water to *yin*; for the upper and the lower, the upper pertains to *yang* and the lower to *yin*.

5.2.2.2 The Categorization of Things According to *Yin* and *Yang*

Two objects (or phenomena) opposing in quality and two aspects opposing in one object (or phenomenon) can be categorized into either *yin* or *yang* according to their shape, tendency, location, and developmental state (Table 5-1). Generally speaking, the side that bears the properties of being active, dispersing, rising, hot, and bright pertains to *yang*, while the side that bears the properties of being relatively static, astringing, falling, cold, and dim pertains to *yin*. Between heaven and earth, the heaven supposed to be formed by light and clear celestial *qi* pertaining to *yang*, and the earth is formed by heavy and turbid terrestrial *qi* to yin. Between dynamics and statics, dynamic objects of exuberant vitality pertain to *yang*, and

Table 5-1   *Yin* and *Yang* Qualities of Objects and Phenomena

Quality	Space	Time	Season	Temperature	Humidity	Brightness	Weight	Moving States
Yang	Upper Outside	Day	Spring Summer	Hot	Dry	Bright	Light	Ascending Active Excitement Exuberance Outward Gasification
Yin	Lower Inside	Night	Autumn Winter	Cold	Humid	Dark	Heavy	Descending Static Inhibition Decline Inward Condensation

static objects of quiet vitality to *yin*. As for the tendency of substances, the active tendency of gasification pertains to *yang*, and the relatively static tendency of condensation to *yin*. As to the life process, the substance with the functions of propelling, warming, and exciting like *qi* pertains to *yang*, and the substance with the functions of condensing, moistening, and inhibiting like blood pertains to *yin*.

After long-term observation, the ancient Chinese found that water and fire were the most typical contradiction and could be used to represent the objects or phenomena pertaining to *yin* and *yang* due to their characteristics. Water is cold, dim, and downward-moving, and fire is hot, bright and up-flaming. Water and fire are used to signify *yin* and *yang* in *Plain Questions*, which makes the abstract notion of *yin-yang* much easier to be understood.

5.2.2.3 Universality and Relativity of *Yin-yang*

The theory of *yin-yang* is the ancient dualism with the naive idea of materialist dialectics and is the basic method. It guides ideology for ancient Chinese to analyze things and understand the world. *Yin-yang* is characterized of its universality and relativity.

The universality of *yin-yang* lies in the fact that the world is the unity of opposites: *yin* and *yang*. Just as what is said in *Plain Questions*, Chapter 5, "Clear *yang* accumulates upward to form heaven, and turbid *yin* deposits downward to form the earth. Terrestrial *qi* ascends to become cloud, and celestial *qi* becomes rain when it descends." Everything in the universe contains two opposing aspects: *yang* and *yin*, such as day and night, sunny and rainy, hot and cold, dynamic and static. As in the intrinsic character of everything, the interaction of *yin* and *yang* results in the occurrence, development, and change of everything in the cosmos. That is why *Plain Questions*, Chapter 5 states that "*yin* and *yang* are the general law of nature, and are the origin of birth, development, variation and demise of everything."

The relativity of *yin-yang* means that *yin* and *yang* properties are not absolute and unitary. That can be defined in terms of different qualities or aspects of things. *Yin-yang*, an abstract summary of opposing sides of interrelated objects and phenomena, is a variable signifier, whose connotation varies with the signified. For example, *yang* and *yin* can be used to signify various pairs, such as heaven and earth, upper and lower, external and internal, fire and water. Just as what is said in the notes for *Plain Questions* by Wang Bing, "The relationship between the signifier of *yin-yang* and the signified is like that between water and its container, namely, the connotation of *yin-yang* is decided by the specific signified." Besides, the relative *yin* and *yang* properties vary with the change of the standard, such as time, location, and condition (*An Expounding of the Formularies of the Bureau of the People's Welfare Pharmacies*).[80] The relativity of *yin-yang* is shown in the following two aspects.

First, *yin* and *yang* can mutually transform. The maximum effect of one quality will be followed by the transition toward the opposing quality. In other words, once the maximum *yang* aspect has manifest ed (such as the appearance caused by extreme heat in the heat syndrome: feverish face and dry tongue with reddish tip), this will be followed by the transition toward the *yin* aspect (with the appearance of the cold syndrome: aversion to cold and cold limbs).

Second, *yin* and *yang* can be infinitely divided. Since *yin* and *yang* are relative, further dividing *yang* and *yin* into their respective *yin* and *yang* aspects yields four combinations: the *yin* of *yang*, the *yang* of *yang*, the *yin* of *yin*, and the *yang* of *yin*. For example, daytime pertains to *yang* and night to *yin*. Daytime can be further divided into two phases: morning and afternoon. Since *yang-qi* ascends in the morning and descends in the afternoon, morning pertains to *yang* (the *yang* of *yang*) and afternoon to *yin* (the *yin* of *yang*). Similarly, night can be divided into anterior night and posterior night. Since *yin-qi* increases in the anterior night and decreases in the posterior night, anterior night pertains to the *yin* of *yin* and posterior night pertains to the *yang* of *yin*. Therefore, any two correlated objects (or phenomena) in nature can be divided into *yin* and *yang*; any one object (or phenomenon) can be divided into two aspects of *yin* and *yang*; and any aspect of *yin* or *yang* can be further divided into *yin* and *yang*. The phenomenon of opposition and interdependence of things is infinite in the natural world.

5.2.2.4 *Yin-yang* is the Basic Law of Natural Change

Yin-yang theory holds that any one object (or phenomenon) contains the opposing *yin* and *yang* aspects. Since the interaction of *yin* and *yang* is the intrinsic attribute of everything in the cosmos, *yin* and *yang* are regarded as the general law of the motion and change in the natural world by ancient thinkers. Just as what is said in *Plain Questions, Chapter 5: The Principle of Yin-yang Doctrine and Its Relation between Nature and Human Body*, "the movement of *yin* and *yang* produces heaven and the earth, generates seasons as well as day and night, creates the necessities of life for organisms, produces *qi* and blood in the human body; in conclusion, *yin* and *yang* are the origin of everything."

Yin and *yang* play different roles because of their different qualities. It is said in *Plain Questions*, Chapter 5 that *yin* is static and has the function of generating the form of objects, while *yang* is active and has the function of *qi*-transformation. Despite the contrary quality, *yin* and *yang* are necessary in the constitution and the movement of objects; their interaction leads to the occurrence, development, decline, and demise of everything.

5.2.3 Basic Contents of *Yin-yang* Theory

The basic contents of *yin-yang* theory can be expounded from the perspectives of their interaction, opposition, interdependence, wane-wax, and mutual-transformation.

5.2.3.1 *Yin-yang* Interaction

The so-called *yin-yang* interaction refers to such a basic process as *yin-yang* intercourse. It is pointed out in *Yi Zhuan* that *yin-yang* interaction is the essential condition for the generation of all things. "The interaction between descending celestial *qi* and ascending terrestrial *qi* gives rise to the changes of the cosmos" (*Plain Questions*, Chapter 68). In the natural world, descending *yang-qi* and ascending *yin-qi* interact to form a cloud, fog, thunder, lightning, rain, and dewdrop, which generate and nourish all the living things. The intercourse between man and woman gives birth to new life and ensures human reproduction. *Yin-yang* interaction occurs in the process of their movement, where *yin* and *yang* are in a balance. Zhuang Zi had the understanding in *Chuang-tzu Wai Pian·Tian Zi Fang*: "When *yin* descending from heaven and *yang* ascending from the earth meet and reach a state of harmony, everything will be generated."

To sum up, *yin* and *yang* are in constant motion and interact when they meet and reach a state of harmony. This interaction unifies two opposing substances or forces, and leads to the generation and change of nature including human beings.

5.2.3.2 *Yin-yang* Opposition

By *yin-yang* opposition, we mean any two correlated objects (or phenomena) are opposite in quality, or each of them has two opposing aspects: *yin* and *yang*. The opposites struggle, restrain, and repel each other, which makes them united and stays in a relative balance.

All things in the nature are in an opposite balance: upper and lower; left and right; heaven and earth; dynamic and static; outward and inward; ascending and descending; day and night; bright and dark; cold and hot; and water and fire. A dynamic *yin-yang* balance can be obtained through *yin-yang* opposition, which can be either mutual restriction or *yin-yang* wane-wax. For example, four seasons experience the climatic changes of warm, heat, cool, and cold; these seasonal climate features are the result of the mutual struggle and restraint between *yang-qi* and *yin-qi*. Warmth in spring and heat in summer result from the inhibition of the cool and cold *yin-qi* by the ascending *yang-qi*; and cool in autumn and cold in winter result from the inhibition of warm and hot *yang-qi* by ascending *yin-qi*. *Plain Questions*, Chapter 17 states that *yang-qi* ascends gradually and *yin-qi* descends gradually in the forty-five days from the Winter Solstice to the Beginning of Spring; and then *yang-qi* reaches its peak and *yin-qi* is hidden on the Summer Solstice, thereafter *yin-qi* ascends gradually and *yang-qi* descends gradually in the forty-five days from the Summer Solstice to the Beginning of Autumn; and then *yin-qi* reaches its peak and *yang-qi* is hidden on the Winter Solstice. This circle proceeds year by year.

Besides nature, the human body itself is also an organic unity of the opposing *yin* and *yang* in its mutual struggle and restraint. For example, the unity of excitement and inhibition of human function is the result of mutual restraint and repulsion. Excitement (*yang*) dominates the daytime when *yang-qi* is exuberant. That is why we can study and work energetically in the daytime. Inhibition (*yin*) dominates night when *yin-qi* is predominant; it restrains and repels the excitement of human function, and therefore man sleeps at night. Because of the harmony of excitement (*yang*) and inhibition (*yin*) of human function, life activities can be normally maintained.

Yin-yang opposition runs through the whole developmental process of all things, in plants' sprouting, growing, transforming, reaping, and storing, as well as in animals' birth, growth, maturity, aging, and death. Only on the basis of opposition, can the dynamic *yin-yang* balance be maintained, and thus things develop endlessly. When *yin-yang* opposition goes abnormally, the *yin-yang* equilibrium will be destroyed. For example, for two opposites, if one side is too strong, the other will be restrained excessively and become weak; contrarily, if one side is too weak to restrain the other, the latter will become excessively strong.

Besides *yin-yang* opposition, there is another united and complementary relation between *yin* and *yang*, i.e., *yin-yang* interdependence.

5.2.3.3 *Yin-yang* Interdependence

Yin-yang interdependence means that *yin* and *yang* depend on and promote each other, and no one can exist without the existence of the other. For instance, the upper (*yang*) and the lower (*yin*) cannot exist without the other. So do such pairs as heaven and earth, day and night, cold and hot in natural phenomena, left and right, south and north in position, and body and life activity, *zang-fu* organs and their functions, *qi* and blood in the human body. In a word, the existence of one side is the condition for that of the other. *Yi Guan Bian · Yin Yang Lun*[81] believes that "*yin* and *yang* are mutually rooted: *yin* cannot be produced without *yang* and *yang* cannot be generated without *yin*." *Yin-yang* interdependence deeply reveals their inseparability. Specific to the human body, life activities (*yang*) cannot be produced without the body (*yin*), and the body (*yin*) will die without life activities (*yang*). As to *zang-fu* organs (*yin*) and their functions (*yang*), *zang-fu* organs (*yin*) are the material bases for their functions (*yang*); and the latter keeps the former in a normal state. That is why *Plain Questions*, Chapter 5 holds that in the human body, *yin*, the material basis of *yang*, remains inside to support the movement of *yang*; and *yang*, the functional activity of *yin*, stays outside to protect *yin*. This normal interdependent relationship gets the life activities maintained.

However, when the interdependence is destroyed, diseases will occur and even life will be threatened, because under pathological conditions, the deficiency of *yin* or *yang* will bring on the consumption of the other. Specifically, *yin* will be deficient when yang declines to a certain degree, for "*yin* cannot be produced without *yang*," which is called "the impairment of *yang* affecting *yin*." For example, patients suffering prolonged anorexia due to asthenia of spleen-*qi* always have to suffer the insufficiency of blood. The spleen and stomach are the material bases for the acquired constitution, responsible for receiving, digesting, and transforming water and food, and therefore are the sources of *qi* and blood. Asthenic spleen-*qi* (*yang*) fails to transform foods into nutrients in the blood and therefore brings on the deficiency of blood (*yin*). It is called the deficiency syndrome of both *qi* and blood due to "the impairment of *yang* affecting *yin*." Likewise, *yang* will be insufficient when *yin* declines to a certain degree, for "*yang* cannot be generated without *yin*," which is called "the impairment of *yin* involving *yang*." For instance, blood (*yin*) carries *qi* (*yang*); excessive hemorrhage leads to the exhaustion of *qi*, and thus results in a *yang*-asthenia syndrome with the manifestation of cold body and limbs. It is described as the deficiency syndrome of both *qi* and blood due to "the impairment of *yin* involving *yang*." When *yin-yang* interdependence is severely damaged, life will be threatened, for if one side turns too weak to exist, the other side will soon lose the prerequisite of the existence.

The abnormal *yin-yang* interdependence may result in either mutual-impairment of *yin* and *yang*, or the separation of *yin* and *yang*. For one thing, the impairment of one side affects the other and eventually leads to the impairment of both *yin* and *yang*. A case in point is that the declination of the physiological function (*yang*) will cause the deficiency of life substances (*yin*), and vice versa. For another, the unbalanced interdependence will lead to the solitary state of *yin* or *yang*, where things can neither grow nor exist. In the human body, the separation of *yin* and *yang* will cause death.

In short, *yin-yang* opposition and interdependence are the two aspects of the basic relationship between *yin* and *yang*. The former embodies the irreconcilability between *yin* and *yang*, and the latter reflects their inseparability. *Yin* and *yang* are two opposing and, at the same time, complementary aspects of a contradiction entity.

5.2.3.4 *Yin-yang* Wane-wax

Yin-yang wane-wax means that the opposing *yin* and *yang* aspects are not in a static state but in a dynamic equilibrium. Namely, as one aspect declines, the other increases to an equal degree.

Yin-yang wane-wax is caused by *yin-yang* opposition and *yin-yang* interdependence. Wane-wax itself is imbalanced, namely, one aspect of *yin* and *yang* waxes while the other wanes, but generally speaking, at a certain stage and within a certain limitation it maintains a relative balance, otherwise wane-wax will result in the disintegration and extinction of the original things.

Yin-yang wane-wax involves the following two basic forms. One is associated with *yin-yang* opposition: one side of *yin-yang* wanes and the other waxes, namely, one side is weakened and the other is strengthened. The other is relevant to *yin-yang* interdependence: both *yin* and *yang* wane or wax, i.e., both of them are weakened or strengthened.

In terms of *yin-yang* theory, constant wane-wax produces various changes of nature, such as the revolving of the hosts of the heaven, the changes of seasons, the alternation of day and night, and the transformation between substance and function. Take the climatic changes in the four seasons, for example. The climatic change from spring warmth to summer heat is caused by *yang* waxing and *yin* waning, and the climatic change from autumn cool to winter cold results from *yin* waxing and *yang* waning. As is stated in *Plain Questions*, Chapter 17, *yang-qi* gradually ascends through *yang* waxing and *yin* waning in the forty-five days from the Winter Solstice to the Beginning of Spring, so the weather gets warmer and warmer; *yin-qi* gradually rises through *yin* waxing and *yang* waning in the forty-five days from the Summer Solstice to the Beginning of Autumn, and therefore the weather becomes cooler and cooler. The regular wane-wax movement of *yin* and *yang* in four seasons results in the regular changes of climate.

The physiological function of the human body is another case in point. Since man corresponds with nature, the excitement of human function dominates the daytime when *yang-qi* is predominant, and the inhibition of human function dominates night when *yin-qi* is exuberant. *Yang-qi* begins to ascend at midnight and reaches its peak at midday, and correspondingly human function gradually changes from inhibition to excitement in this period, which is called the process of "*yin* waning and *yang* waxing"; *yang-qi* declines gradually while *yin-qi* flourishes gradually from midday to midnight, and correspondingly human function changes from excitement to inhibition, which is called the process of "*yang* waning and *yin* waxing." Therefore, in the daytime and at night, excitement and inhibition are always in an absolute imbalance in which one wanes while the other waxes, but they maintain a relative balance in the overall time from daytime to night. Then let's take substance and function of the human body, for another example. The human body carries out various functions by consuming nutrients, which is called "*yin* waning and *yang* waxing;" the human body generates and transforms all kinds of nutrients by expending energy, which is called the process of "*yang* waning and *yin* waxing." The former is dissimilation (*yang*) and the latter assimilation (*yin*), which maintains a relative balance on the whole in the normal human body. This is called "balance between *yin* and *yang*" by the ancient Chinese. Therefore, the wane-wax and the *yin-yang* balance are the essential conditions to maintain normal physiological activities.

Yin-yang wane-wax is manifested in both *yin-yang* opposition and *yin-yang* interdependence. Take *qi* and blood for example. *Qi* (*yang*) can produce blood (*yin*), which is the reason why *qi* deficiency always leads to blood inadequacy and finally results in the deficiency syndrome of both *qi* and blood, which is called "waning of both *yin* and *yang*." On the contrary, replenishing *qi* can promote the generation of blood and restore both *qi* and blood, which is named "waxing of both *yin* and *yang*." Take substance and function, for another example. Function (*yang*) results from the movement of substance (*yin*). There is no motionless substance in the cosmos, and accordingly there is no substance without function and no function without a substance's movement. A sound physiological function depends on the abundance of such substances as *qi*, blood, body fluids, and essence, and vice versa. Some physiological functions are affected due to being restrained or obstructed, which will lead to the insufficiency of *qi*, blood, body fluids, and essence; the overconsumption of such physiological substances also results in the deficient physiological functions. These are called "waning of both *yin* and *yang*." The affected physiological functions can be restored through regulation, which will also restore the insufficient substances, and vice versa. These are called "waxing of both *yin* and *yang*." Consequently, "waning or waxing of both *yin* and *yang*" is the manifestation of *yin-yang* interdependence.

Yin-yang wane-wax and balance accord with the basic law that movement is absolute while stillness is relative, and thus wane-wax is absolute while balance is relative. The absolute movement and relative stillness are intercomponent, i.e., a relative balance is maintained in the absolute wane-wax and the absolute wane-wax exists in a relative balance. Everything develops and changes in the process of the absolute wane-wax and relative balance.

Yin-yang wane-wax is a quantitative result of *yin-yang* movement. If wane-wax is maintained in a proper amount, *yin* and *yang* will stay in a relative balance. Otherwise, it will damage the relative balance and result in predomination or declination of either *yin* or *yang*.

5.2.3.5 *Yin-yang* Transformation

Under certain conditions, *yin* and *yang* will turn to the opposite, namely, *yin* will change into *yang* and *yang* into *yin*. For one thing, the inherent foundation of the mutual transformation is their mutual interdependence, for one exists with the other as the precondition.

5.2 The Theory of Yin-yang

For another, the internal cause of *yin-yang* transformation is their wane-wax. When the quantitative change caused by their wane-wax exceeds a certain limitation, it will consequentially lead to the qualitative change, the *yin-yang* transformation. For example, since extreme *yin* can turn into *yang* and extreme *yang* into *yin*, extreme cold (*yin*) leads to heat (*yang*), and extreme heat (*yang*) to cold (*yin*). This causes seasonal variation.

There are two essential ways of *yin-yang* transformation: gradual change and drastic change. Gradual change means that in the wane-wax process, *yin* gradually transforms into *yang* by *yang* waxing and *yin* waning; *yang* gradually changes into *yin* by *yin* waxing and *yang* waning. Seasonal change and the alternation of day and night are the typical examples. Drastic change refers to the fact that when the quantitative wane-wax reaches its extreme, a qualitative mutual transformation occurs abruptly and quickly. A good case in point is that in the hot summer, a sudden heavy shower, the result of *yang* (heat) waxing and *yin* (cool) waning reaching its peak, brings down the heat and leads to cool.

In the natural world, *yin-yang* transformation is manifested as the incessant alternation of four seasons: The cold winter (*yin*) transforms into the warm spring (*yang*), and the hot summer (*yang*) transforms into the cool autumn (*yin*).

In the human life process, the *yin* and *yang* aspects of the human body are also mutually transforming. In terms of the relationship between nutrients and *qi*-transformation, the human body maintains the normal life activities by transforming nutrients (*yin*) into the function of *qi*-transformation (*yang*) ceaselessly. On the other hand, it transforms foods into the required nutrients through the normal *qi*-transformation of *zang-fu* organs. Such a mutual transformation between substance and function is progressive and fluctuates with the fluctuation of *yin-yang* wane-wax. In the daytime, since *yin* wanes and *yang* waxes in catabolism, a lot of nutrients are consumed and transformed into the function of *qi*-transformation, which is the process of *yin* transforming into *yang*; at night since *yang* wanes and yin *waxes* in anabolism, nutrients digested and absorbed through the normal *qi*-transformation are stored in the body, which is the process of *yang* transforming into *yin*. These incessant *yin-yang* transformations guarantee the normal life activities.

In the developmental process of diseases, under certain conditions, the mutual-transformations may occur between exterior syndrome and interior syndrome, cold syndrome and heat syndrome, deficiency syndrome and excessive syndrome, as well as *yin* syndrome and *yang* syndrome. For instance, high fever, reddish complexion, irritability and rapid-strong pulse are the symptoms of the syndrome of pathogenic heat in the lungs. They are *yang* syndrome, heat syndrome, and excessive syndrome. However, when the disease goes to a severe stage where the extreme pathogenic heat seriously consumes vital energy, it will change into the syndrome of *yang* depletion immediately, whose symptoms are pale complexion, cold limbs, dispiritedness, and faint pulse, which pertains to *yin* syndrome, cold syndrome, and deficiency syndrome. This syndrome variation is the transformation from *yang* to *yin*. Take asthma, for another example. Cough and asthma, whitish and thin sputum, no thirst, light-colored tongue with whitish coating, and taut pulse are symptoms of the cold syndrome of asthma. Invaded by pathogenic cold again, *couli* of the human body is closed due to cold stagnation, which results in the heat syndrome of asthma, whose symptoms are asthma and hoarse breath, yellowish and thick sputum, thirst, reddish tongue with yellowish coating, and rapid pulse. This change of syndrome is the transformation from *yin* into *yang*.

In summary, the basic contents of *yin-yang* theory include *yin-yang* interaction, opposition, interdependence, wane-wax, and transformation, in which wane-wax is a process of quantitative change and mutual-transformation is a qualitative one. The following is the summary of *Yin-yang* theory (Table 5-2).

Note: Taijitu

Interaction, opposition, interdependence, wane-wax, and mutual-transformation between

Table 5-2　Yin-Yang Theory

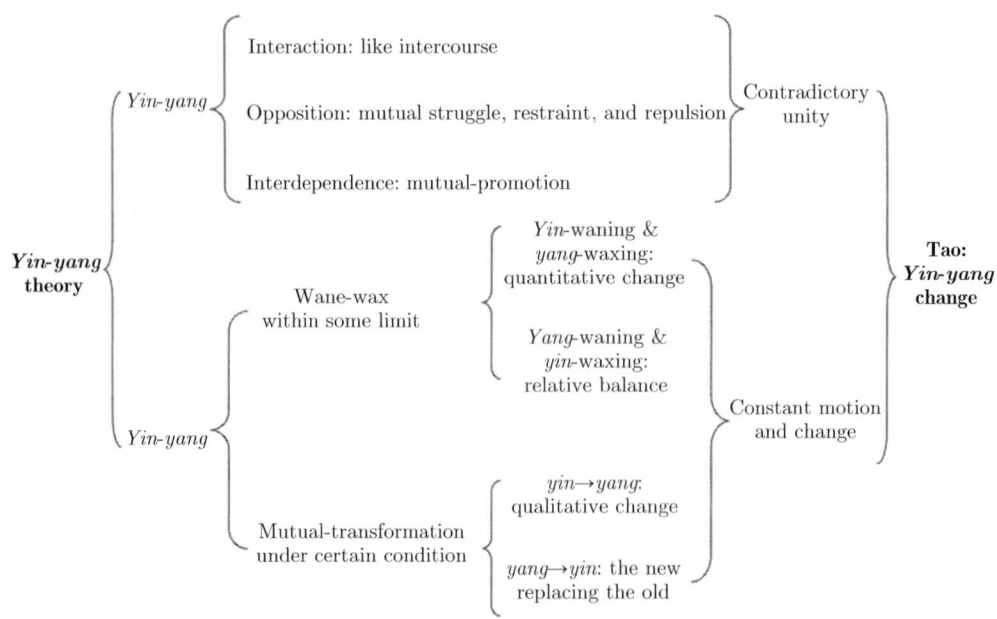

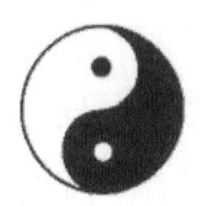

Yin-yang theory	Yin-yang	Interaction: like intercourse	Contradictory unity	**Tao: Yin-yang change**
		Opposition: mutual struggle, restraint, and repulsion		
		Interdependence: mutual-promotion		
	Yin-yang	Wane-wax within some limit	Yin-waning & yang-waxing: quantitative change	Constant motion and change
			Yang-waning & yin-waxing: relative balance	
		Mutual-transformation under certain condition	yin→yang: qualitative change	
			yang→yin: the new replacing the old	

Figure 5-1　Taijitu

yin and yang are dialectically interrelated. Interaction, opposition, and interdependence means yin-yang opposition and coexistence, while wane-wax and mutual-transformation stresses the yin-yang change. Taijitu (Figure 5-1) visually generalizes the dialectical relations mentioned above. The big circle in the schematic diagram represents *Taiji*, i.e., primordial qi, whose movement produces yin and yang, and then the motion of yin and yang generates all things in nature. *Yi Zhuan·Xi Ci* states that the motion of *Taiji* generates yin and yang, whose movement gives birth to the natural phenomena in four seasons, such as spouting in spring, growing in summer, reaping in autumn, and storing in winter, with which all things change. The white part in the left side of diagram denotes yang and the black part in the right side represents yin, which coexist in *Taiji*. There is a small white round that symbolizes yang in the black part, which means that yang is the origin of yin; a small black round that signifies yin exists in the white part, which shows that yin is the root of yang. The two opposite parts in the big circle form an annular graph that symbolizes the unceasingly rotary wane-wax and mutual-transformation between yin and yang with primordial qi as basis. *Diagram annotation of Classified Canon*[82] holds that yin and yang that result from *Taiji* can turn to each other, in which yin transforms into yang by the motion of yin-qi, and yang changes into yin through the condensation of yang-qi. Yin-yang wane-wax and mutual-transformation creates a boundless universe.

5.2.4　The Application of *Yin-yang* Theory in TCM

Yin-yang doctrine has been applied widely and flexibly since it was introduced into the medical field. It not only becomes the cornerstone for ancient physicians to construct the theoretical system of TCM, but also runs through every aspect of clinical practice. It facilitates our understanding about the histological structure, physiological functions, and pathological changes of the human body, and guides the clinical diagnosis and treatment.

5.2.4.1　Explanation of Man's Physical Structure

The human body is an organic unity of opposition. All the tissues and organs are organi-

5.2 The Theory of Yin-yang

cally interrelated and can be divided into two opposite parts in terms of *yin* and *yang*.

First, various parts of the human body can be categorized into *yin* and *yang* in terms of their location: the exterior pertains to *yang* while the interior to *yin*; the upper pertains to *yang* while the lower to *yin*; the back pertains to *yang* while the abdomen to *yin*; the left pertains to *yang* while the right to *yin*; the lateral sides of four limbs pertains to *yang* while the medial sides to *yin*; the head to *yang* while the feet to *yin*; the chest to *yang* while the abdomen to *yin*; the upper limbs to *yang* while the lower limbs to *yin*.

Second, *zang-fu* organs and tissues can be divided into *yin* and *yang*. The internal *zang-fu* organs pertain to *yin*, while the external five constituents (tendons, vessels, muscles, skin, and bones) to *yang*. Speaking of *zang-fu* organs, five *zang*-organs pertain to *yin* for they store essence, while six *fu*-organs to *yang* for they digest foods and discharge waste. As to five *zang*-organs, for one thing, according to the location, the heart and lungs pertain to *yang* for they are located in the chest above the diaphragm, while the liver, the spleen, and kidneys pertain to *yin* for they are located in the abdominal cavity below the diaphragm. For another, according to the attribute of Five Elements, the heart pertains to the *yang* of *yang* because it pertains to fire in Five Elements and corresponds with summer; lungs pertain to the *yin* of *yang* because they pertain to metal and correspond with autumn; the liver pertains to the *yang* of *yin* because it pertains to wood and corresponds with spring; kidneys pertain to the *yin* of *yin* because they pertain to water and correspond with winter; and the spleen pertains to the supreme *yin* of *yin* because it pertains to the earth and corresponds with late summer.

Third, meridians and collaterals can also be classified into *yin* and *yang*. In terms of meridians, those that run along the medial side of four limbs pertain to *yin* for they are affiliated to five *zang*-organs (*yin*), while those that run along the lateral side of four limbs pertain to *yang* for they are affiliated to six *fu*-organs (*yang*). Concerning collaterals, those that are located in viscera and the deep layer of four limbs pertain to *yin* because the internal pertains to *yin*, while those in the skin and the superficial layer of four limbs pertain to *yang* because the external pertains to *yang*.

In a word, the categorization of the physical structure of the human body into *yin* and *yang* is mainly based on the location, the functional characteristics of *zang-fu* organs, and the attributes of Five Elements. It is not only the simple generalization and contrast of different anatomical parts, but also shows the inherent functional features of *zang-fu* organs and tissues (Table 5-3).

Table 5-3 Categorization of the Histological Structure of the Human Body according to *Yin* and *Yang*

	Body Parts			Histological Structure				
Yang	External	Upper	Back	Lateral Side of Four Limbs	Skin and Hair	Six Fu-organs	Six Yang Meridians of Hand and Foot	Qi
Yin	Internal	Lower	Abdomen	Medial Side of Four Limbs	Tendons and Bones	Five Zang-organs	Six Yin Meridians of Hand and Foot	Blood

5.2.4.2 Explanation of Man's Physiological Function

Yin-yang theory holds that man's physiological function depends on *yin-yang* contradictory unity. Substance (*yin*) and function (*yang*) is a contradictory unity of *yin-yang*, because the performance of physiological functions depends on the movement of such substances as *qi*, bloods, and body fluids, whose metabolism in turn relies on the functional activities of the related viscera. Such a relation is the result of *yin-yang* interdependence and *yin-yang* wane-wax.

Take the physiological function of the *qi*-transformation, for example. The intrinsic form of life activities and the basic characters of life existence are the *qi*-transformation, whose basic styles are ascending, descending, going out, and coming in. Though *yang* ascending and *yin* descending are the inherent nature of *yin-yang*, there are still *yang* descending and *yin* ascending for the *yin-yang* movement. Specifically, both *yin* and *yang* can be respectively subdivided into *yin* and *yang*, and therefore under normal conditions, the *yin* of *yang* descents and the *yang* of *yin* ascents, which make partial *yang* descending and *yin* ascending possible. Since *yin* and *yang* are opposite but unified, ascending and descending as well as going out and coming in are opposing and complementary. The normal life activities depend on such normal *qi*-transformation, otherwise diseases will occur.

Another case is man's respiratory function. Expiration (*yang*) and inspiration (*yin*) are opposite but interdependent. There will be no inspiration without expiration and vice versa. In one breath, expiration is the process of *yang* waxing and *yin* waning, and inspiration is the opposite. Expiration turns into inspiration when it reaches its peak, and vice versa. The conversion from expiration to inspiration and that from inspiration to expiration form a respiratory cycle, whose relative equilibrium is achieved by their wane-wax and transformation.

As to respiratory frequency, the aspect exciting respiratory function and accelerating breath pertains to *yang* and the opposite aspect to *yin*. The regular breath is the result of *yin-yang* balance. When a man sleeps at night, his breath experiences *yin* waxing and *yang* waning, in which *yin* is relatively dominant, so the respiratory frequency slows down; when a man acts in the daytime, his breath undergoes *yang* waxing and *yin* waning, in which *yang* is relatively predominant, and thus the respiratory frequency is higher than that at night. When a man does labor work or intense sports, *yang-qi* is hard to be inhibited by *yin*, for "movement produces *yang*," and so breathing accelerates in a short pant; when a man stops to rest, ever excited *yang-qi* is restrained by *yin*, and then *yin* and *yang* return to a relative balance for "stillness generates *yin*." Thus, it can be seen that within a certain limitation, the normal human body has the automatic adjusting capability to keep *yin* and *yang* in a relative equilibrium.

Besides, human metabolism, heart beat, pulse, body temperature, limb movement, *zang-fu* activity, and so on can also be reasonably explained with *yin-yang* theory, i.e., *yin-yang* opposition, wane-wax, mutual-transformation, and relatively equilibrium.

In addition to inside *yin-yang* activities, humans are also affected by the *yin-yang* changes of the outside world. Namely, the physiological functions of the human body have to adapt to *yin-yang* changes such as seasonal alternation and the day-night shift. For instance, in the daytime (*yang*) a man is predominated by *yang-qi* and is active, and the metabolism is dominated by dissimilation; at night (*yin*) a man is predominated by *yin-qi* and sleeps, and the metabolism is dominated by assimilation. Similarly, in spring and summer, *yang-qi* of the human body ascends for *yang* waxing and *yin* waning; in autumn and winter, *yang-qi* is hidden for *yin* waxing and *yang* waning.

Generally speaking, the human body is an entity constituted by the opposite *yin* and *yang* of various levels. Opposition, interdependence, and relative balance maintained through *yin-yang* wane-wax and transformation can account for a man's vital activities and the unified man-nature relationship. If the relative equilibrium between *yin* and *yang* in the body is damaged, a man will get sick; if *yin* and *yang* separate, a man will die.

5.2.4.3 Explanation of Man's Pathological Changes

Only when the pairs of the internal and the external, the upper and the lower, substance and substance, function and function, as well as function and substance in the body, are kept in relative harmony, can the normal physiological activities be maintained and thus can a man keep healthy. Otherwise diseases occur.

The Classic of Internal Medicine divides the disease causes into *yin* and *yang*. For one thing, etiology can be generally categorized into exogenous pathogenic factors, and endogenous pathogenic factors. The former, such as wind, cold, summer-heat, and dampness, pertains to *yang*, for they can invade the human body from the outside and impair *yang* in the body surface to cause the exogenous exterior syndrome. The latter, like improper diet, improper living conditions, overstrain, excessive sexual activity, and emotional upset, pertains to *yin*, for they can directly damage the activity of visceral *qi* and impair *yin* in the viscera to cause endogenous interior syndrome. For another, both exogenous pathogenic factors and endogenous pathogenic factors can be further divided into *yin* and *yang*. For the exogenous pathogenic factors (mobile pathogenic winds) (*yang*) tend to attack the upper parts of the body such as the head and face, bringing on their pathological changes; sticky and stagnant pathogenic dampness (*yin*) tends to attack the lower parts such as the feet and legs, leading to their pathological changes; pathogenic summer-heat and fire (*yang*) can cause heat syndrome, leading to fever, thirst, and insomnia; stagnated pathogenic cold (*yin*) can bring about cold syndrome, causing aversion to cold, diarrhea, and pain in muscles and joints. As to the endogenous pathogenic factors, excessive emotional changes pertain to *yin* for they can damage the activity of visceral *qi*. Different emotional stimulations, however, can be subdivided into *yin* and *yang*, for they impair different internal organs. Excessive anger pertains to *yin*, for it tends to impair the viscera which pertain to *yin* like the liver, and cause their pathological changes; excessive joy pertains to *yang*, for it tends to damage the viscera which pertain to *yang* like the heart, resulting in their pathological changes. In conclusion, due to different *yin* or *yang* properties of the pathogenic factors and different pathogenic features, the locations of diseases and syndromes are varied.

The occurrence, development, and change of diseases are the states of relative predominance or declination of *yin* or *yang* resulting from abnormal *yin-yang* wane-wax caused by the struggle between vital energy and pathogenic factors. In terms of *yin-yang* theory, diseases are the results of the invasion of pathogenic factors, which causes the struggles between pathogenic factors (*yang*) and *yin*-fluid, and those between pathogenic factors (*yin*) and *yang-qi*. The struggles lead to the *yin-yang* imbalance, with various pathological manifestations like relative predominance, relative declination, mutual consumption, mutual transformation, and mutual rejection between *yin* and *yang*. That's why TCM always takes pathogenic factors and vital energy, and *yin-yang* balance into great consideration in generalizing the pathological changes of disease.

- **Relative Predominance of *Yin* or *Yang***

Relative Predominance of *yin* or *yang* is a pathological change due to excessive increase of *yin* or *yang* caused by the invasion of exogenous pathogenic factors which pertain to *yin* or *yang*. Increasingly predominant *yin* or *yang* turns into a pathogenic factor and will inevitably inhibit or damage the other, making it decline. Just as what is said in *Plain Questions*, Chapter 5, "*yin* and *yang* in the human body must always be kept in balance. The predominance of *yin* will cause *yang* disease and the exuberance of *yang* will lead to *yin* disorder."

For one thing, *yang* exuberance will bring about heat syndrome. For example, the invasion of pathogenic summer-heat will make *yang-qi* hyperactive, leading to high fever, sweating, thirst, reddish complexion, and rapid pulse. With the progression of the disease, pathogenic factors which pertain to *yang* consume *yin*-fluid, bringing on thirst. So it is stated that "*yang* exuberance will lead to *yin* disorder," which means that the exuberance of *yang* impairs *yin*-fluid of the human body.

For another, the predominance of *yin* will result in cold syndrome. For instance, the intake of cold food or drink will make *yin-qi* predominant, leading to abdominal pain, diarrhea, light-colored tongue with a white coating, and deep pulse. With the progression of the disease, pathogenic factors which pertain to *yin* impair *yang-qi*, bringing on a cold body and limbs. So it is stated that "*yin* predominance will cause *yang* disease," which means that the predominance of *yin* will inevitably damage the *yang-qi* of the human body.

The above two are caused by the invasion of exogenous pathogenic factors into the body, and are "exuberance of pathogenic factors leading to excess syndrome."

- **Relative Deficiency of *Yin* or *Yang***

Relative deficiency of *yin* or *yang* refers to the pathological changes, where *yin* or *yang* declines below the normal level. In general, it mainly results from the insufficiency of *yin*-fluid or *yang-qi*. The relative declination of one side decides that it cannot restrain the other, and will inevitably lead to the relative predominance of the other side.

First, *yang* deficiency leads to cold syndrome. Deficient *yang-qi* fails to restrain *yin* and makes *yin* relatively exuberant, bringing on cold syndrome, like pale complexion, aversion to cold, cold limbs, lassitude, spontaneous sweating, and faint pulse.

Second, *yin* deficiency leads to heat syndrome. Deficient *yin*-fluid fails to restrict *yang*, and renders *yang* relatively predominant, and thus heat syndromes appear. For example, the *yin* deficiency caused by a prolonged disease can result in hectic fever, night sweat, feverish sensation in the chest, palms and soles, dryness of mouth and tongue, thready and rapid pulse.

The above two are caused by the deficiency of vital energy due to the attack from exogenous pathogenic factors or the insufficiency of *qi*, blood, and *yin* or *yang* of the human body itself. It is called "deficiency of vital energy leading to asthenia syndrome" in TCM.

- ***Yin-yang* Mutual Impairment**

Yin-yang mutual impairment refers to the pathological changes where asthenia of *yin* or *yang* develops to a certain degree and then leads to the insufficiency of the other. According to the principle of *yin-yang* interdependence, the deficient *yin* or *yang* fails to promote the transformation of the other, and therefore in the end the other side will also be insufficient. Namely, "the impairment of *yang* affects *yin*" or "the impairment of *yin* involves *yang*." These two pathological changes will finally result in the syndrome of *yin-yang* deficiency.

Yin-yang mutual impairment is another manifestation of the relative deficiency of *yin* or *yang*. The only difference lies in that, at the primary stage of the relative deficiency of *yin* or *yang*, the deficient *yin* or *yang* fails to restrain the other and thus makes the other relatively predominant. *Yin-yang* mutual impairment means that when the deficiency of one side develops to a certain extent, the other will get insufficient for the lack of the independence from the former. Thereafter, it is the mutual impairment on the basis of *yin-yang* independence.

Clinically, in order to distinguish "heat syndrome caused by *yang* exuberance" from "heat syndrome due to *yin* deficiency," TCM calls the former Heat of Excess Type and the latter Heat of Deficiency Type; similarly, "cold syndrome caused by *yin* exuberance" is called Cold of Excess Type and "cold syndrome due to *yang* deficiency" is called Cold of Deficiency Type. The syndrome caused by "*yang* impairment affecting *yin*" is deficiency-syndrome, in which Cold of Deficiency Type is primary and Heat of Deficiency Type is secondary; the syndrome due to "impairment of *yin* involving *yang*" is deficiency syndrome where Heat of Deficiency Type is primary and Cold of Deficiency Type is secondary.

- **Mutual-transformation and Mutual-rejection between *Yin* and *Yang***

Mutual-transformation and mutual-rejection between *yin* and *yang* are the pathological

5.2 The Theory of Yin-yang

changes due to the overabundance of *yin* or *yang*. Mutual-transformation means that *yang* syndrome transforms into *yin* syndrome or vice versa. The property of the disease changes in mutual-transformation. By mutual-rejection, we mean that symptoms of cold syndrome appear in heat syndrome and symptoms of heat syndrome appear in cold syndrome. They are the pathological changes of "extreme *yang* like *yin*" and "extreme *yin* like *yang*." Different from mutual-transformation, the property of the disease does not change in mutual-rejection.

In terms of mutual-transformation, cold syndrome and heat syndrome may transform into each other, when they reach their peaks due to delayed treatment or erroneous therapy. That is so-called "extreme cold leading to heat, and extreme heat to cold," and "excessive *yang* turning into *yin*, and excessive *yin* into *yang*." For example, patients suffering acute Spring Warm disease have the clinical manifestations of heat syndromes, such as high fever, reddish complexion, stiffness and pain of the head and neck, and rapid pulse. If treatment is delayed or the wrong therapy is carried out, the disease may develop to the extreme, with the symptoms of cold syndrome: sudden descent of body temperature, cold limbs, pale complexion, mental confusion, and extreme faint pulse. This is the transformation of heat syndrome into cold syndrome.

As to mutual-rejection, the predominant side of *yin* or *yang* stays inside and drives the deficient side outside, and thus the two sides of *yin* and *yang* cannot coordinate with each other, leading to the pathological changes of "cold syndrome with pseudo-heat symptoms" and "heat syndrome with pseudo-cold symptoms." The former is caused by "predominant *yin* rejecting *yang*"; the latter results from "exuberant *yang* repelling *yin*."

Mutual-transformation and mutual-rejection between *yin* and *yang* are essentially two pathological changes, differing in that the former involves the essential change of *yin* or *yang* properties, while the latter does not.

The following are the diagrams of relative predominance or deficiency of *yin* or *yang* (Figures 5-2 to 5-7).

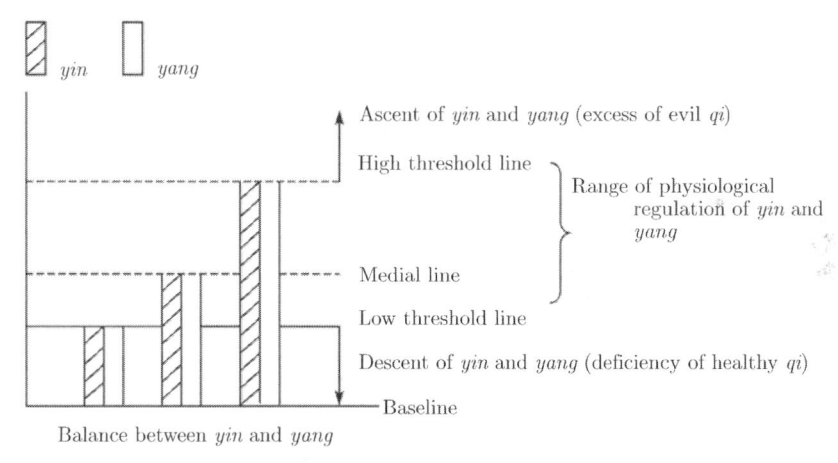

Figure 5-2 Diagram of Balance between *Yin* and *Yang*

5.2.4.4 Guiding Clinical Diagnosis

In terms of TCM's *yin-yang* theory, diseases are the results of *yin-yang* imbalance. Clinically, no matter how complicated and changeable diseases are, they can be analyzed with *yin-yang* theory. Therefore, the categorization of *yin* and *yang* is the key to diagnosis. Ancient physicians emphasize that "experts in diagnosis always start with the differentiation between *yin* syndrome and *yang* syndrome by observing the complexion and palpating the

Yang-exuberance   Yin-exuberance

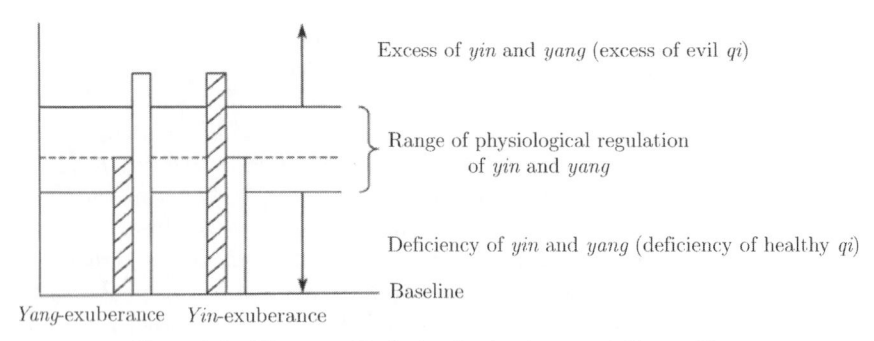

Figure 5-3   Diagram of Relative Predominance of *Yin* or *Yang*

Yang-deficiency   Yin-deficiency

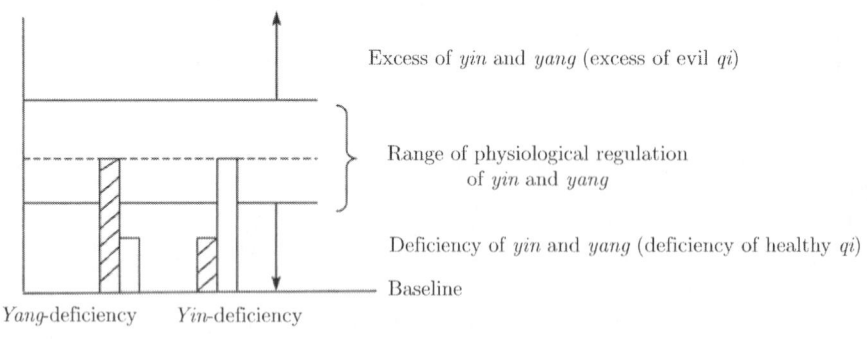

Figure 5-4   Diagram of Relative Deficiency of *Yin* or *Yang*

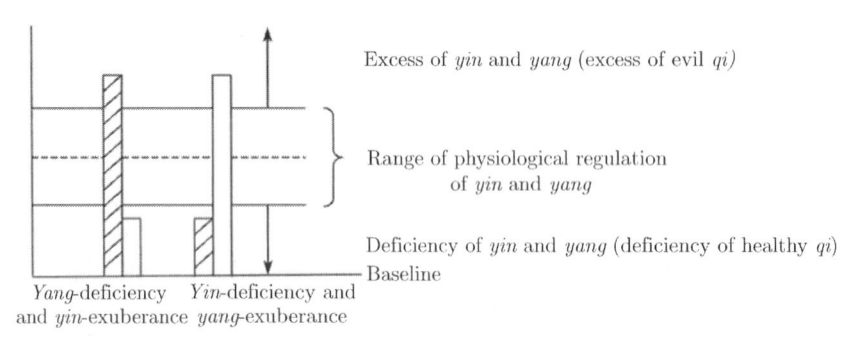

Yang-deficiency   Yin-deficiency and
and yin-exuberance   yang-exuberance

Figure 5-5   Diagram of Relative Predominance or Deficiency of *Yin* or *Yang*

Predominance of both *yin* and *yang*

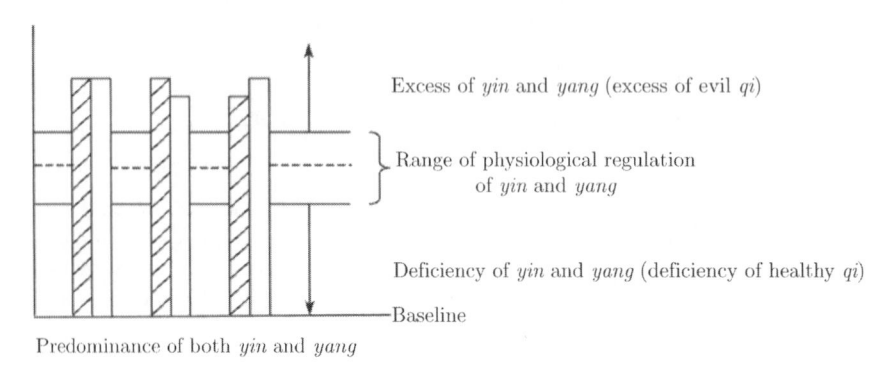

Figure 5-6   Diagram of Predominance of Both *Yin* and *Yang*

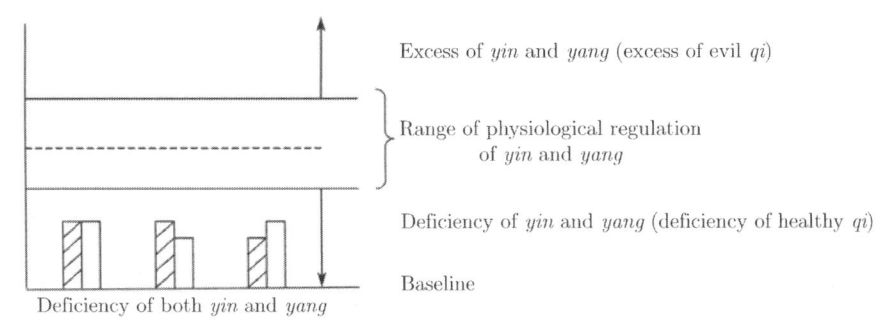

Figure 5-7 Diagram of Deficiency of Both *Yin* and *Yang*

pulse." Differentiation helps to generalize the basic attribute of the whole syndrome and analyze the concrete symptoms and physical signs.

Syndromes are usually differentiated from the aspects of *yin* and *yang*, external and internal, cold and heat, as well as deficiency and excess. It is the "Eight-principle Syndrome Differentiation." Among them, *yin* and *yang* are regarded as the general ones. According to such a gradation, external syndrome, excess syndrome, and heat syndrome pertain to *yang* syndrome, while others to *yin* syndrome. *Yin-yang* theory is also used to differentiate visceral syndromes. For example, syndromes of five *zang*-organs pertain to *yin* and syndromes of six *fu*-organs to *yang*. Clinically, to differentiate the syndrome is to differentiate *yin* and *yang*.

In addition, complexion, voice, symptoms, and pulse can be analyzed in terms of *yin* and *yang*, too. Bright complexion pertains to *yang*, while grayish complexion to *yin*; husky respiration and sonorous voice pertain to *yang*, while weak, respiration and low and weak voice to *yin*; fever, thirst, and constipation pertain to *yang*, while aversion to cold, no thirst, and loose stool to *yin*. In terms of pulse position, *Cun*-pulse pertains to *yang* while *Chi*-pulse to *yin*; as to pulse dynamics, rising pulse pertains to *yang* while falling pulse to *yin*; as for pulse frequency, rapid pulse pertains to *yang* while slow pulse to *yin*; speaking of the emerging site of pulse, floating pulse pertains to *yang* while sunken pulse to *yin*; with regard to pulse shape, large, full, and slippery pulse pertain to *yang*, while uneven, thin, and small pulse to *yin*. Obviously, *yin-yang* is the guiding principle in diagnosis.

5.2.4.5 Guiding Clinical Treatment

Clinically, *yin-yang* theory is used to decide the therapeutic principles and to generalize the properties of drugs.

- **Deciding Therapeutic Principles**

Since the occurrence and development of diseases result from *yin-yang* imbalance, the general therapeutic principle is to regulate *yin* and *yang*, i.e., to restore their relative balance by supplementing the deficiency and reducing the excess.

Therapeutic principles for Relative Predominance of *Yin* or *Yang* are as follows. Since Relative Predominance of *Yin* or *Yang* may bring on excess syndrome (whose basic pathogenesis is the exuberance of pathogenic factors), the treatment must follow the principle: "treating excess syndrome with purgation." Specifically, the Heat Syndrome of Excess Type due to the exuberance of pathogenic factors (*yang*) should be treated by clearing away heat with herbs of cold and cool nature, which is called "treating heat syndrome with cold therapy." The Cold Syndrome of Excess Type due to the exuberance of pathogenic factors (*yin*) should be treated by eliminating cold with herbs of warm and heat nature, which is termed as "treating a cold syndrome with warm therapy." The progression of Relative Predominance may lead to the impairment of *yin*-fluid or *yang-qi*, which should be treated by eliminating pathogenic factors in combination with deficiency-supplementing therapy, i.e., combination therapy of clearing away heat and nourishing *yin*, or combination therapy of eliminating cold and strengthening *yang*.

Therapeutic principles for Relative Deficiency of *Yin* or *Yang* are as follows. Since Relative Deficiency of *Yin* or *Yang* may bring on deficiency syndrome whose basic pathogenesis is the insufficiency of *yin* or *yang*, its therapeutic principle is that "deficiency syndrome should be treated with nourishing therapy." Specifically, the Heat Syndrome of Deficiency Type due to *yin* insufficiency should be treated not by clearing away heat with herbs of cold and cool nature, but by nourishing *yin*, which is termed as "treating *yang* disease from *yin* aspect" in *Plain Questions*. The Cold Syndrome of Deficiency Type due to *yang* insufficiency should be treated not by eliminating cold with herbs of warm and heat nature, but by strengthening *yang*, which is called "treating *yin* disease from *yang* aspect" in *Plain Questions*.

Since *yin* and *yang* are interdependent, the insufficiency of one side may affect the other and then result in the deficiency syndrome of both *yin* and *yang*, and should be treated by nourishing both *yin* and *yang*. The deficiency syndrome of both *yin* and *yang* caused by the insufficiency of *yang* should be treated mainly by strengthening *yang* with the consideration of *yin*; the deficiency syndrome of both *yin* and *yang* due to the insufficiency of *yin* should be treated mainly by nourishing *yin* with the consideration of *yang*. In this way, *yin* and *yang* can generate and promote each other, which is helpful for their restoration.

- **Guiding Clinical Acupuncture and Moxibustion Therapy**

The important twelve meridians of the human body can be grouped into six pairs. Each pair is in an internal-external relation, and pertains to *yin* and *yang*, respectively. *Yin* meridians pertain to *zang*-organs and connect *fu*-organs, while *yang* meridians do the opposite. The twelve meridians are connected with each other like a loop, which not only makes the human body an organic integrity, but also makes disease transmission along meridians possible. Therefore, diseases in a certain viscus are usually treated by acupuncturing the meridian pertaining to the viscus itself, assisted by acupuncturing the meridian connecting the viscus and the proximal meridian. Likewise, the treatment of diseases that are located in the upper parts of the body can be assisted by acupuncturing the lower parts, and vice versa; diseases on the left sides can be cured with the help of acupuncturing the right parts, and vice versa; pathogenic factors in the *yang* meridian can be cured by acupuncturing the *yin* meridian, and vice versa.

- **Generalization of the Properties of Chinese Medicinal Herbs**

Yin-yang theory can also explain the properties of the Chinese medicinal herbs. Clinically, the preconditions to satisfactory treatment are the choice of correct therapeutic principles based on correct diagnosis, and the selection of proper Chinese medicinal herbs in terms of their properties.

Chinese medicinal herbs are of four properties of cold, cool, warm, and hot, where cold and cool pertain to *yin* while warm and hot to *yang*. Chinese medicinal herbs of cool or cold nature such as *Gypsum Fibrosum*, *Radix Scutellariae*, *Fructus Gardeniae*, and *Radix Rehmanniae* can be used to treat heat syndrome; those of warm or hot nature like *Ramulus Cinnamomi*, *Fructus Evodiae*, *Rhizoma Alpiniae Officinarum*, and *Fructus Psoraleae* can be used to treat cold syndrome. Here we should notice that although the property of cold-dispelling herbs and that of *yang*-invigorating ones are all warm and hot, their efficacies are not the same; though the property of heat-clearing herbs and that of *yin*-nourishing ones are all cool and cold, but their efficacies are different. Therefore, it is necessary to select the proper herbs according to the concrete conditions of diseases besides properties.

Chinese medicinal herbs are of five flavors: acrid, sweet, sour, bitter, and salty. Actually, some herbs are not as distinct as any of the above five flavors, and they are of bland or acerbic flavor. Acrid, sweet, and bland flavors pertain to *yang*, while others to *yin*, and thus the functions of herbs with acrid or sweet, mild tastes mainly pertain to *yang*, while the functions mostly to *yin*. Since various herbs possess diverse properties and flavors, due consideration of these properties will be helpful in choosing herbs.

Chinese medicinal herbs tend to act on the body in four directions: upward, downward, outward, and inward. In TCM, they are specifically named ascending, descending, floating, and sinking. Ascending and floating pertain to *yang* while descending and sinking to *yin*. The herbs with the following functions pertain to *yang*: elevating *yang* and expelling superficial pathogenic factors, expelling wind and dissipating cold. The herbs with the following functions pertain to *yin*: purgation, clearing away heat, promoting urination, tranquilizing mind, promoting digestion to remove food retention, and descending adverse flow of *qi* to stop vomiting.

In brief, only when Relative Predominance or Deficiency of *Yin* and *Yang* is clearly differentiated, can correct therapeutic principles be decided and proper herbs be selected.

- **Guiding Health Maintenance and Disease Prevention**

Health maintenance and disease prevention are important components in TCM. TCM holds that prevention to some extent is more important than treatment.

To maintain health, man has to follow the law of *yin-yang* variation, for man is closely related to nature whose seasonal changes influence man's physiological functions. Since the liver corresponds with the sprouting of spring, the heart to the growing of summer, lungs to the reaping of autumn, and kidneys to the storing of winter, human beings should pay attention to the maintenance of the liver and the heart in spring and summer and attach importance to the maintenance of the lung and the kidney in autumn and winter.

Health maintenance involves the prevention of exogenous pathogenic factors, the regulation of emotions, and the balance of diet and daily life. *Plain Questions* says that "to maintain health, man should adapt himself to climatic changes of four seasons, keep tranquil mind, and reside in a safe and comfort place. In such a way, *yin* and *yang* of the human body are regulated to maintain health."

5.3 The Theory of Five Elements

The theory of Five Elements, like *yin-yang* theory, is one important philosophical doctrine in ancient China. It holds that the natural world derives from such five basic substances as metal, wood, water, fire, and earth, whose interpromotion and interrestraint produce the motion, change, and prevalent association of the natural world. The theory has a great impact on the formation and development of TCM.

5.3.1 The Formation and Development of the Theory of Five Elements

The theory of Five Elements originated from Chinese cognitions about five directions, 3000 years ago. In the Shang dynasty (1600-1046 B.C.), people took their residential area as the center to differentiate the east, west, south, and north. There is some record about the rain and wind from different directions in the oracle bone script: The directions of the wind and rain vary with seasons and climates, and therefore decide people's agricultural production: cultivating in spring, growing in summer, harvesting in autumn, and storing in winter. Such a close association between space and time lays a foundation for ancient Chinese to extend the concept of Five Elements to a more general classification of natural phenomena.

In Spring-Autumn Period, the theory of "five materials" emerged after the theory of "five directions." It is firstly recorded in *Zuo Commentary* that the nature produces five kinds of indispensable materials which people depend on to live, i.e., metal, wood, water, fire and earth: metal and wood are used to make tools; water and fire are used to cook food; and earth ensures the growth of all things. *On Leud States· Zheng* termed five materials the most basic substances constituting the universe.

The notion "Five Elements" was first brought up in *Shang Shu*[83]: the natural phenomena are classified into water, fire, wood, metal and earth according to their properties and flavors. Water is characterized by moistening and flowing downward; fire is characterized by flaming upward; wood is characterized by being flexed and extended; metal is characterized by being changed in form, and earth is the place where crops grow. As to their flavors, things of water property are salty, fire bitter, wood sour, metal pungent and earth sweet. This excerpt not only explains the properties and flavors of Five Elements, but also shows their corresponding relations. Five properties do not belong to the five concrete substances themselves alone, they are the high generalization of all the things about their attributes. Thereafter the notion of "Five Elements" becomes an abstract philosophical concept, used to analyze all the things in the natural world.

TCM has been greatly influenced by the philosophy of Five Elements. *Plain Questions· Tian Yuan Ji Da Lun* holds that the movement and change of everything in the world must follow the law of Five Elements and the universe goes by the doctrines of inter-promotion, inter-restraint, over-restraint and counter-restraint among Five Elements.

5.3.2 The Characteristics of Five Elements

The characteristics of Five Elements are the rational generalization of the features of Five Elements themselves. It is not only the theoretical basis to analyze the properties of all things but also the basic law to study their interrelationships. Therefore, it has more extensive and abstract meanings than Five Elements themselves.

- **The Characteristic of Wood**

The trunks of trees grow upward and straight; their exuberant branches stretch upward and outward. Therefore, the element of wood is characterized of flexing and extending, growing, and freedom. Things or phenomena of these properties pertain to wood.

- **The Characteristic of Fire**

When fire is burning, its flame flies upward, and its light and heat spread outside. Therefore, the element of fire is characterized of flaming up, warmth, ascending and brightness. Things or phenomena of these properties pertain to fire.

- **The Characteristic of Earth**

Earth is called the mother of everything, for all things grow in the earth: it is where minerals store, vegetation grows, crops produce, and living things exist. Therefore the element of earth is characterized by cultivation, reception, fosterage and harvest. Things or phenomena of these properties pertain to earth.

- **The Characteristic of Metal**

Metal is hard, depurating and astringing. It can be made into sharp weapons and tools, so the element of metal is characterized by being changeable in form, depurative, astringent, and descensive. Therefore, things or phenomena of these properties pertain to metal.

- **The Characteristic of Water**

Water is characterized by softness, coolness, moistening, and flowing downward, so things or phenomena of these properties pertain to water.

One thing is worth noting. The characteristics of Five Elements originate from the five concrete substances but transcend them. For example, when the terms of wood, fire, earth, metal, and water are used to elucidate the structures and functions of *zang-fu* organs of the human body, they refer to the properties of the specific organs. A specific case is that lungs pertaining to metal do not mean that they are made of metal but that like the element of metal, lungs are of the property of dispersion, descent, depuration, and astringency.

5.3.3 Categorization and Deduction of Things in Terms of Five Elements

The theory of Five Elements classifies things into five categories according to their properties. For example, if a thing is similar to wood in property, it pertains to wood; if it is similar to fire in property, it pertains to fire. Accordingly, all the things in the natural world can be analyzed into five categories at varied levels. In TCM, histological structure, physiological and pathological phenomena of the human body are classified in terms of the properties of Five Elements, and thus formulate a *zang*-organ centered system of Five Elements. The macro system of Five Elements in the natural world and the micro system of Five Elements in the human body are interrelated, and things that pertain to the property of the same element are interrelated, interpromoting and interrestricting. There are two specific ways to categorize things in an analogy with Five Elements: direct analogy, and indirect inference and induction.

- **Direct Analogy**

Direct analogy can be made between specific things and the attributes of Five Elements.

First, direction is categorized in terms of Five Elements. East pertains to wood for it is where the sun rises, having the property of rising up like wood; west pertains to metal, for it is where the sun sets, having the properties of depuration, astringency, and descent like metal; south pertains to fire, for it is hot in the south, having the properties of warmth, ascending, and brightness like fire; north pertains to water, for it is cold in the north, similar to the coolness of water.

Second, seasons can also be categorized in the properties of Five Elements. Spring, characterized by the resuscitation of all things, is similar to wood in property and thus pertains to wood. Summer, characterized by hot weather and the luxuriant growth of all things, is similar to fire in property, and thus pertains to fire. The rainy season in summer is called late summer, which is characterized by high temperature and humidity, which is beneficial to the maturity of fruits, and similar to the earth in property, and therefore pertains to the earth. Autumn, characterized by the decline of all things, is similar to metal in property, and that is why autumn pertains to metal. Winter, characterized by cold weather and animal hibernation, is similar to water in property, and for this reason winter pertains to water.

Third, *qi*, transformation, color, and the like all can be classified according to the properties of wood, fire, earth, metal, and water, which is easier to be understood in the Chinese natural conditions. China lies in the North Temperate Zone, and climates vary with directions. In spring, the gentle wind mostly blows easterly, trees sprout and the earth is decorated with green, so east, spring, wind, warm, germination, and green are related. Similarly, in the hot summer, wind mostly blows southerly, the sun shines like red fire, plants and animals fully grow, and thus south, summer, heat, red, and growth are related. In cool and dry autumn, leaves begin to fall due to westerly winds, crops are harvested and the earth turns white, and therefore west, autumn, dry, cool, white, and reaping are related. In cold winter, the brisk northerly winds and the icy earth force creatures to hide themselves, and the short day and long night make sunlight weak, so north, winter, cold, black, and storing are related.

Fourth, various *zang-fu* organs, tissues, and organs are categorized in terms of the properties of Five Elements. The liver governs *shu xie* (dredging and regulating), so it pertains to wood; the heart warms the whole body, and thus pertains to fire; the spleen carries and transforms food nutrients, and therefore pertains to earth; lungs function to depurate and descend, and they pertain to metal; kidneys control the metabolism of body fluid, so pertain to water.

In the above aspects, direct categorization of things according to the properties of Five Elements is made on the basis of only some partial properties of things. Therefore, it has certain limits, which can be overcome by indirect inference and deduction.

- **Indirect Inference and Deduction**

By indirect inference and deduction, we mean when one thing is categorized as one property, other related things are also categorized into the same category.

Based on long-term observation and clinical practice, ancient Chinese doctors classify the human body into the categories of wood, fire, earth, metal, and water through inference and deduction. For example, dampness in late summer tends to impair the spleen, bringing on poor appetite, chest oppression, nausea and vomiting, greasy taste in the mouth, lassitude of the muscles; the spleen prefers sweet, and modest sweet taste invigorates the spleen but superabundant sweet taste obstructs the function of the spleen and stomach. Therefore, interrelated late summer, dampness, sweet, yellow, spleen, stomach, mouth, and muscles all pertain to earth.

Various histological structures and functional activities can be categorized into five functional systems centering around five *zang*-organs according to the properties of Five Elements (Table 5-4). These are the taxonomic basis for the establishment of *zang-xiang* theory.

Each element in Five Elements, as the table shows, is externally related to the things and phenomena in nature and internally relative to various viscera, tissues, organs, functions, and pathological changes. Take the element of wood for example. Wood, characteristic of flexing and extending, has the property of growth, development, and freedom. In spring, the warm weather, easterly winds, resuscitation of all things, propagation of grass and trees, verdant earth and sour fruits are similar to the properties of wood, so "east" in five directions, "spring" in five seasons, "wind" in five kinds of *qi*, "germination" in five transformations, "wheat" in five grains, "sour" in five flavors, and "green" in five colors all pertain to wood. In the human body, the liver prefers freedom to stagnation, so liver pertains to wood. In physiology, the liver and gallbladder are of internal and external relation, and the liver opens into the eyes, governs the tendons, and is associated with the emotion of anger; in pathology, the dysfunction of the liver will bring on susceptibility to rage, and the insufficiency of liver-blood fails to nourish the tendons, leading to spasm. Thus, the tissues, organs, physiological functions, and pathological changes which are closely related to the liver also pertain to wood in Five Elements.

Zang-organs can be expounded in terms of the properties of Five Elements. The liver governs the ascending *qi* of spring and prefers freedom to stagnation, so it pertains to wood; the heart dominates the growing *qi* of summer and can warm the whole body, and thereby pertains to fire; the spleen controls the transforming *qi* of late summer and governs the transformation and transportation of food nutrients, and thus pertains to earth; lungs dominate the descending *qi* of autumn and govern descent, and therefore pertain to metal; kidneys dominate the storing *qi* of winter and store essence, and so pertain to water.

Second, the categorization elucidates the systematization of the human body. The human body is divided into five physiological systems centering around five *zang*-organs. And the relationship between the physiological and pathological changes of five physiological systems can be explained with the laws of the interpromotion and interrestraint among Five Elements.

Third, categorization based on Five Elements expounds the unity of man and nature. According to the theory, nature and the human body are two similar structural systems,

5.3 The Theory of Five Elements

Table 5-4 The Categorization of the Human Body and Nature according to the Properties of Five Elements

Five Smells	Five Notes	Five Fu-Organs	Five Sensory Organs	Five Colors	Five Flavors	Five Grains	Five Transformations	Five Kinds of qi	Five Seasons	Five Directions	Five Elements
Foul	Jue	Gallbladder	Eye	Green	Sour	Wheat	Germination	Wind	Spring	East	Wood
Empyreumatic	Zhi	Small Intestine	Tongue	Red	Bitter	Broomcorn Millet	Growth	Heat	Summer	South	Fire
Fragrant	Gong	Stomach	Mouth	Yellow	Sweet	Proso Millet	Transformation	Dampness	Late Summer	Center	Earth
Fishy	Shang	Large Intestine	Nose	White	Pungent	Rice	Reaping	Dryness	Autumn	West	Metal
Rancid	Yu	Urinary Bladder	Ear	Black	Salty	Bean	Storing	Cold	Winter	North	Water

Five Zang Organs					Five Spirits Constituents	Five Emotions	Five Sounds	Five Kinds of Liquids	Five Activities	Five Elements
Liver				Tendon	Ethereal Soul	Anger	Shout	Tear	Hold	Wood
Heart				Vessel	Spirit	Joy	Laugh	Sweat	Worry	Fire
Spleen				Muscle	Mind	Contemplation	Sing	Saliva	Keck	Earth
Lung				Skin & Hair	Corporeal Soul	Grief	Cry	Snivel	Cough	Metal
Kidney				Bone	Will	Fear	Groan	Spittle	Tremble	Water

not only with the corresponding elements related horizontally, but also related in the change of elements vertically.

5.3.4 Fundamental Contents of the Theory of Five Elements

The basic contents of the theory of Five Elements can be generalized into interpromotion, interrestraint, overrestraint and counterrestraint.

5.3.4.1 Interpromotion and Interrestraint among Five Elements

It is interpromotion and interrestraint that guarantee the ecological balance and physiological balance.

- **Inter-promotion**

One element in the Five Elements promotes another in certain order: wood promoting fire, fire promoting earth, earth promoting metal, metal promoting water, and water promoting wood, which form a circle. Each of Five Elements is connected with others for it is both "being promoted" and "promoting," just like the relation of mother and child. The one promoting others is called "mother," while the one promoted is the "child" (*Classic of Medical Problems*). Analogically, the one promoting fire is wood, so wood is the mother of fire; the one promoted by fire is earth, and thus earth is the child of fire. The rest can be deduced by analogy like Figure 5-8.

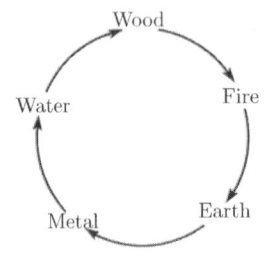

Figure 5-8 The Order of the Interpromotion among Five Elements

Interpromotion among Five Elements shows that different things or various parts of the same thing can be mutually generated and promoted. The reason why one element can promote another is that the former possesses the foundation and potential to promote the latter. Namely, wood can generate fire, for it is of warm nature, and it produces fire when it is drilled; similarly, fire can produce earth, for when things are burned with fire, ashes come out and become earth; earth can generate metal, for earth accumulates to a hill, where metal stores; metal generates water, for it is of depuration, astringency, and descent nature, which are the conditions water appear; water can generate wood, for with water living things grow, which is the nature of wood.

- **Interrestraint**

One element in Five Elements restrains another in certain orders: wood restraining earth, earth restraining water, water restraining fire, fire restraining metal, and metal restraining wood, which form a circle (Figure 5-9). Each of Five Elements relates with others for it is both "restrained" and "restraining," namely it is both a "dominator" and a "submitter" (*The Classic of Internal Medicine*). Take fire for example. Water can restrain fire, so water is the dominator of fire; fire can restrain metal, and thus metal is the submitter of fire. The rest can be deduced by analogy. Therefore, the interrestraint among Five Elements actually means that one element restrains its submitter in Five Elements.

5.3 The Theory of Five Elements

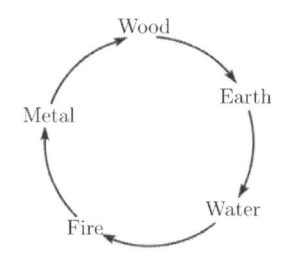

Figure 5-9 The Order of the Interrestraint among Five Elements

Thanks to the interrestraint among Five Elements, the balance among Five Elements can be maintained, for what is restrained is what is excessive. When excessive extending is restrained by water, wood becomes steady; when excessive heat is restrained, fire turns stable; when excessive dampness is restrained, earth keeps lenitive; when excessive coolness is restrained, metal does not shrink; and when excessive water is restrained by earth, there is no flood.

- **The Relationship between Interpromotion and Interrestraint**

Each of Five Elements is characterized by such relationship as "being promoted," "promoting," "being restrained," and "restraining" (Figure 5-10). Although "being promoted" and "promoting" belong to interpromotion among Five Elements, there is still interrestraint in interpromotion. For instance, wood is promoted by water and promotes fire, in which fire is restrained by water. "Being restrained" and "restraining" belong to interrestraint among Five Elements, but there is still interpromotion in interrestraint. For example, wood is restrained by metal and restrains earth, in which earth can promote metal. Therefore, intergeneration and interrestriction are inseparable. Without promotion, nothing can grow and develop; without restraint, there will be no way to prevent harm caused by the excessive development of things. Consequently, restraint in promotion and promotion in restraint keep things develop harmoniously. As to the system of Five Elements, various parts are closely related, in which change of each part will affect others and will be affected and restrained by the integrity of Five Elements. No two parts are in static balance because of their interpromotion and interrestraint. Each of Five Elements is in a relative dynamic equilibrium due to the relationships of "promoting," "being promoted," "restraining," and "being restrained." With interpromotion and interrestraint, the normal changes of climates occur, and ecological and physiological balances are maintained.

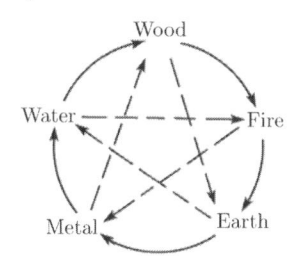

Figure 5-10 Interpromotion and Interrestraint among Five Elements

5.3.4.2 Overrestraint and Counterrestraint among Five Elements

Overrestraint and counterrestraint among Five Elements refer to the abnormal interrestraint when normal interpromotion and interrestraint are damaged.

- **Overrestraint**

Overrestraint refers to an abnormal state where one element excessively restrains another.

There are two causes for overrestraint. One is that one element becomes too powerful compared with the element it normally restrains, and the restrained is excessively weak. Take wood for example. Under normal circumstances, wood restrains earth. If wood is too powerful, earth will be excessively restrained by wood and become weaker, which is known as "wood overrestraining earth" (Figure 5-11).

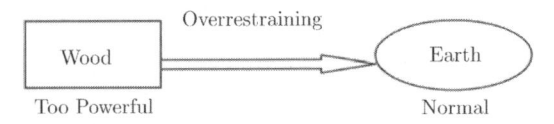

Figure 5-11 Wood Overrestraining Earth

The other cause for overrestraint is that one element becomes too weak to match the element restraining it. For instance, wood normally restrains earth. However, if earth becomes weak, it will be excessively restrained by wood and become weaker, which is known as "earth being excessively restrained by wood" (Figure 5-12).

Though the order of overrestraint is the same as that of interrestraint, they are essentially different. Interrestraint is a normal restraint relation among Five Elements, while overrestraint is an abnormal result from one element's excessive power or weakness (Figure 5-13).

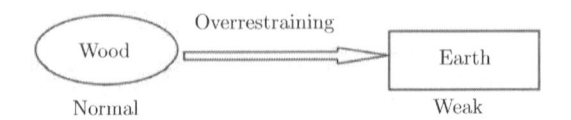

Figure 5-12 Earth Being Excessively Restrained by Wood

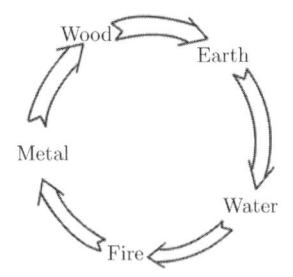

Figure 5-13 The Order of the Overrestraint among Five Elements

- **Counterrestraint**

Counter-restraint is an abnormal state where one element restrains what normally restrains it. There are two reasons for counterrestraint. One is that one element of Five Elements becomes too powerful and thus turns to restrain its dominator. The other is that one element becomes weak and is restrained by its submitter. Take wood for example. Normally, metal restrains wood and is the dominator of wood. If wood becomes too powerful, it will reversely restrain metal, which is termed as "wood counterrestraining metal" (Figure 5-14).

Normally, wood restrains earth and earth is called the submitter of wood. If wood becomes too weak to restrain earth, it will be restrained by earth, which is called "earth counter-restraining wood" (Figure 5-15).

5.3 The Theory of Five Elements

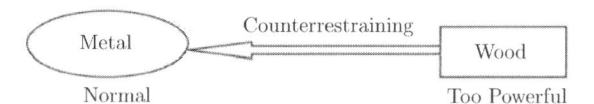

Figure 5-14 Wood Counterrestraining Metal

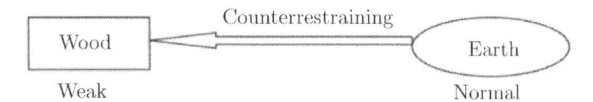

Figure 5-15 Earth Counterrestraining Wood

The order of counterrestraint is opposite to that of interrestraint, and they are essentially different. Interrestraint is a normal restraint relationship among Five Elements, while counterrestraint is an abnormal state for one element becomes too powerful or too weak (Figure 5-16).

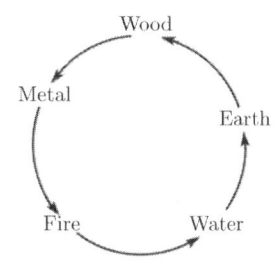

Figure 5-16 The Order of the Counterrestraint among Five Elements

Both overrestraint and counterrestraint are abnormal state where the relative coordination is destroyed (Figure 5-17). Overrestraint means that one element in Five Elements excessively restrains its submitter, and counterrestraint means that one element in Five Elements reversely restrains its dominator.

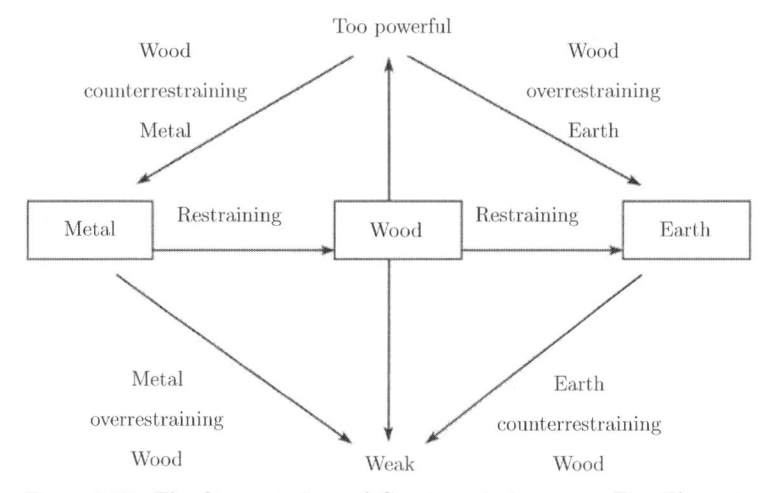

Figure 5-17 The Overrestraint and Counterrestraint among Five Elements

Overrestraint and counterrestraint are the two sides of one thing, and thus can be analyzed together. As *Plain Questions*, Chapter 67 states, "When one element among Five Elements becomes too powerful, it over-restrains its submitter and counter-restrains its dominator; when one element becomes excessively weak, it will be overrestrained by its dominator and counterrestrained by its submitter." For instance, wood becomes too powerful to be restrained by metal, and in turn, excessively restrains earth that it normally restrains, which is called "over-restrain." At the same time, because of excessive power, wood may counterrestrain its dominator metal; on the contrary, if wood becomes too weak, it will be overrestrained by metal and counter-restrained by its submitter earth.

5.3.4.3 The Regulation of Five Elements

The regulation of Five Elements means that within certain limits, the system of Five Elements reregulate the abnormal changes like overrestraint and counterrestraint to restore the new balance through its interpromotion and interrestraint. When one element becomes superabundant, it will be pacified by its dominator through interrestraint, thus it will be weakened in restraining its submitter to restore the original balance.

Take wood, for example. If wood becomes too powerful, it will overrestrain earth and earth will be weakened in restraining water, and thus water is superabundant in restraining fire and fire will be weakened in restraining metal. As a result, metal becomes powerful to make the system of Five Elements restore the normal balance (Figure 5-18). Contrarily, if wood becomes weak, it will be weakened in restraining earth and earth become powerful to restrain water excessively, and therefore water will be powerless to restrain fire and fire become excessively powerful to restrain metal. Consequently, metal becomes too weak to overrestrain wood and wood gradually recovers, which makes the system of Five Elements come back to balance (Figure 5-19).

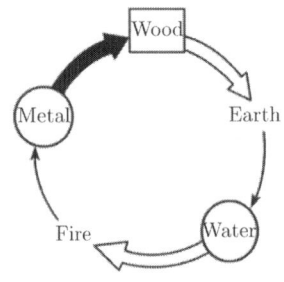

Figure 5-18 Restoration of Wood When It Is Too Powerful

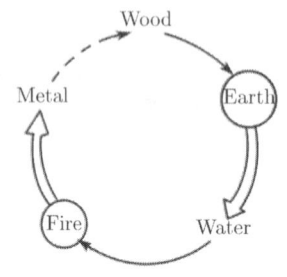

Figure 5-19 Restoration of Wood When It Is Weak

Regulation occurs in the whole system. Without it, the superabundance or weakness of any element will lead to disequilibrium of the whole system. *Plain Questions*, Chapter

5.3 The Theory of Five Elements

68 states that "the hyperactivity of one element in Five Elements will bring about harm, which will be eliminated through the interrestraint among Five Elements." Accordingly, interrestraint is not only the key to maintain normal states of the system but also the intrinsic basis to restore the balance.

To sum up, interpromotion and interrestraint maintain the relative balance of Five Elements, or produce new equilibriums, whereby things develop and change unceasingly. When the enhancement or weakness of any element exceeds certain limits, abnormal states like overrestraint and counterrestraint will break the relative equilibrium of Five Elements. Medically, interpromotion and interrestraint are manifested as physiological phenomena, while overrestraint and counterrestraint are manifested as pathological ones. This chart below is the summary of the basic contents of the interrelationship among Five Elements (Table 5-5).

Table 5-5 Basic Contents of the Interrelationship among Five Elements

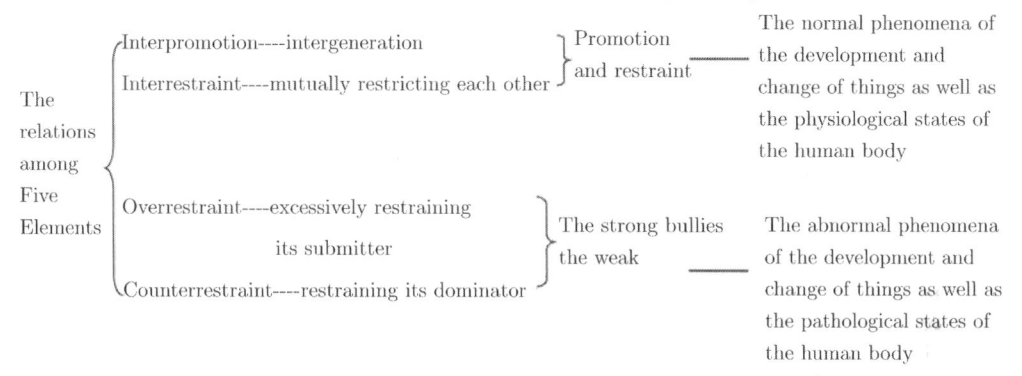

The relations among Five Elements			
Interpromotion----intergeneration	Promotion and restraint		The normal phenomena of the development and change of things as well as the physiological states of the human body
Interrestraint----mutually restricting each other			
Overrestraint----excessively restraining its submitter	The strong bullies the weak		The abnormal phenomena of the development and change of things as well as the pathological states of the human body
Counterrestraint----restraining its dominator			

5.3.5 Application of the Theory of Five Elements in TCM

The theory of Five Elements can be applied to TCM to expound the properties of and interrelation between viscera, meridians, and collaterals. It can also shed light on various physiological functions, pathological phenomena, and thus guide clinical treatment.

5.3.5.1 Explanation of the Physiological Functions and Interrelation of *Zang-fu* Organs

With Five Elements as an analogy, the physiological functions of tissues and organs can be generalized into five physiological systems centering around five *zang*-organs. The theory can also be used to expound the physiological relations between *zang*-organ and *fu*-organ in the same system.

First, TCM pairs five *zang*-organs with the corresponding Five Elements and explains the physiological functions of five *zang*-organs according to the attributes of Five Elements.

The liver pertains to wood, for it governs *shu xie* (dredging the routes and regulating the movement of *qi*) and therefore prefers freedom to stagnation, accordant with the wood's attributes of flexing, extending, and developing. The heart pertains to fire, for it dominates blood circulation and pumps blood to warm the body, accordant with the fire's attributes of flaming up. The spleen pertains to earth, for it transforms water and food to nourish *zang-fu* organs and four limbs, accordant with the earth's attributes of generating all things. Lungs pertain to metal, for, accordant with the attribute of metal, they have the function of depuration. Kidneys pertain to water, for they store essence and manage water metabolism, accordant with water's attributes of moistening, moving downward, and storing.

Second, TCM also elucidates the intrinsic relationships among their physiological functions with the theory of interpromotion and interrestraint of Five Elements.

In terms of interpromotion of Five Elements, the liver promotes the heart corresponding to wood's promoting fire, because the liver stores blood and helps the heart to dominate blood circulation; the heart promotes the spleen corresponding to fire's promoting earth, for only when the heart functions normally, can the spleen be nourished by blood to transport and transform food nutrients and generate blood; the spleen promotes lungs corresponding to earth's promoting metal, because the spleen transports, and transforms food nutrients that will be absorbed and transformed into sufficient qi and blood to nourish the lungs, and it promotes the lungs to dominate qi; lungs promote kidneys corresponding to metal's promoting water, for the lungs depurate and descend qi to help the kidneys absorb qi; the kidneys promote the liver corresponding to water promoting wood, for the essence in kidneys is transformed into blood that will be stored in the liver.

In terms of the interrestraint of Five Elements, kidneys restrain the heart corresponding to water's restraining fire, for kidney-*yin* can assist the heart to control the hyperactivity of heart-*yang*; the heart restrains lungs corresponding to fire's restraining metal, because the warmth of heart-*yang* can prevent lung-*qi* from excessively depurating and descending; lungs restrain the liver corresponding to metal's restraining wood, for lung-*qi* depurates and descends to prevent liver-*yang* from excessively ascending; the liver restrains the spleen corresponding to wood's restraining earth, because liver-*qi* can relieve the stagnation of spleen-*qi*; the spleen restrains kidneys corresponding to earth's restraining water, for the spleen transports and transforms water to prevent kidney water from flooding.

Third, for the correspondence between five *zang*-organs and Five Elements, the human body can be categorized into five basic systems centering around five *zang*-organs.

The liver (wood) system is dominated by the liver, composed of the tissues, organs, and their functional activities that pertain to wood. Its *fu*-organ is the gallbladder, the constituent is tendons, the external manifestation is nails, the orifice is eyes, liquid is tears, and emotion, is anger.

The heart (fire) system, with heart as the center, consists of the tissues, organs, and their functional activities pertaining to fire. Its *fu*-organ is the small intestine, the constituent is vessels, the external manifestation is the face, the orifice is the tongue, liquid is sweat, and emotion is joy.

The spleen (earth) system, with the spleen as the leader, is made up of the tissues, organs, and their functional activities that pertain to earth. Its *fu*-organ is the stomach, the constituent is muscles, the external manifestation is the lip, the orifice is the mouth, liquid is saliva, and emotion is contemplation.

The lung (metal) system, led by the lung, is composed of the tissues, organs, and their functional activities pertaining to metal. Its *fu*-organ is the large intestine, the constituent is skin, the external manifestation is body hair, the orifice is the nose, liquid is snivel, and emotion is grief.

The kidney (water) system, centered on the kidney, is formed by the tissues, organs, and their functional activities that pertain to water. Its *fu*-organ is the urinary bladder, the constituent is the bones, the external manifestation is hair, the orifice is ears, liquid is spittle and, emotion is fear.

Fourth, the hierarchy of the five *zang*-organ systems, as well as their interpromotion and interrestraint can also be expounded with the theory of Five Elements. The human body is an organic integrity of a multilayered structure. The longitudinal structure of five systems are five *zang*-organs, six *fu*-organs, five constituents, five sense organs, and five external manifestations to the five systems, which are of the corresponding properties of Five Elements (Figure 5-20). Meanwhile, its horizontal structure consists of the liver, heart, spleen, lung, and kidney systems. They form a crisscross structure, which establishes the theoretical foundation for "judging the interior from the exterior."

5.3 The Theory of Five Elements

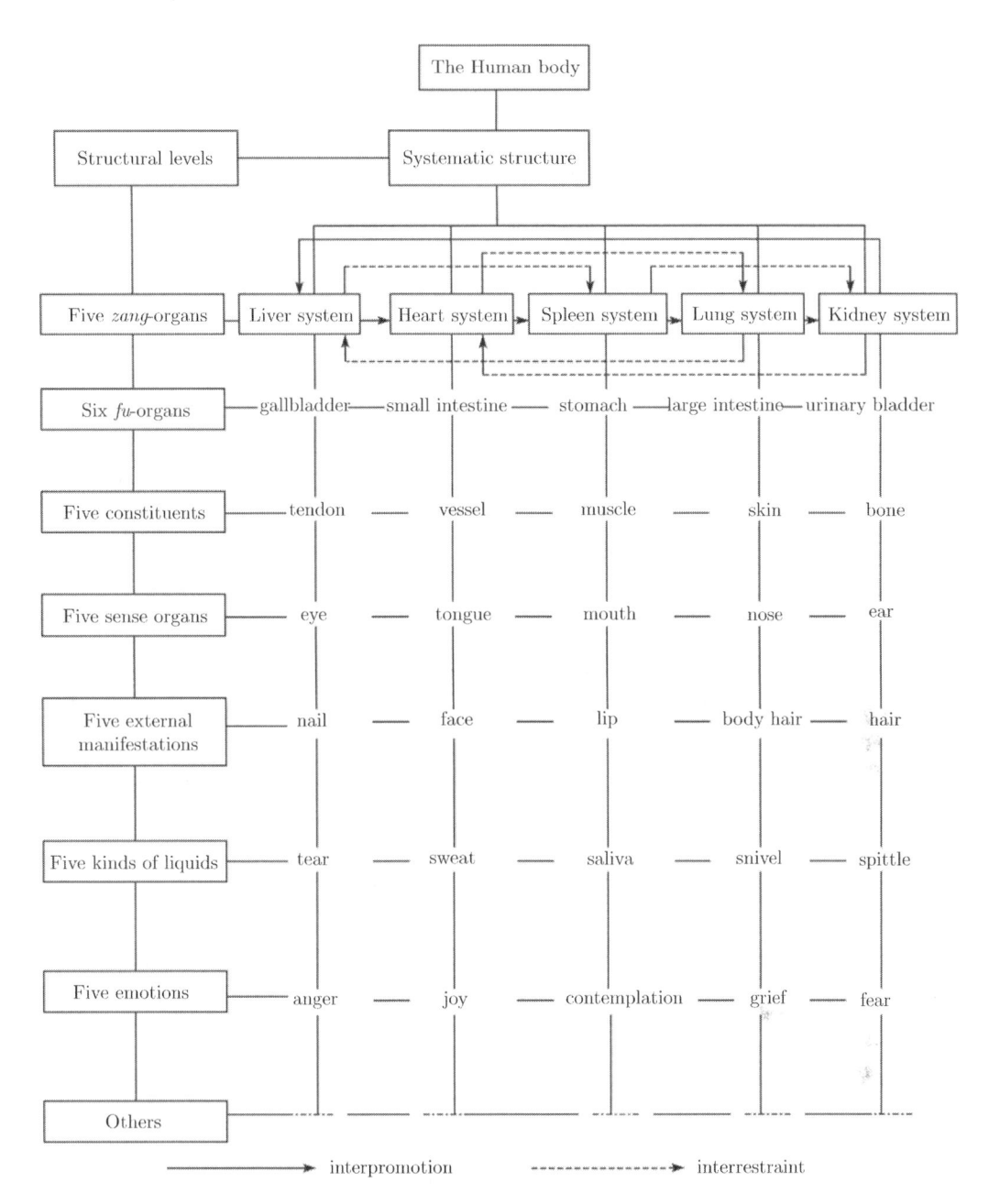

Figure 5-20 Model of the Structural System of Five Elements

Fifth, the theory of Five Elements can also be used to explain the relationship between man and nature. It classifies all things in the nature into the categories of wood, fire, earth, metal, and water; analyzes their movements and changes with the motional law of Five Elements; and investigates the influence of these changes on the human body with the analogy of Five Elements. *Plain Questions*, Chapter 5 states that "East generates wind, wind generates wood, wood generates sour, sour generates the liver, the liver generates tendons, and the liver opens into the eyes and is related to anger in emotion. South generates heat, heat generates fire, fire generates bitter, bitter generates the heart, the heart generates vessels, and the heart opens into the tongue and is related to joy in emotion. The central region generates dampness, dampness generates earth, earth generates sweet, sweet generates the spleen, the spleen generates muscles, and the spleen opens into the mouth and is related to contemplation in emotion. West generates dryness, dryness generates metal, metal generates pungent, pungent generates lungs, lungs generate skins and body hair, and lungs open into the nose and are related to grief in emotion. North generates cold, cold generates water, water generates salty, salty generates kidneys, kidneys generate bones, and kidneys open into the ears and are related to fear in emotion."

The theory of Five Elements shows that man's physiological and emotional changes have something to do with the change of nature. TCM uses the perspective of "correspondence between man and nature" to explain the effects of five directions, five seasons, five kinds of *qi*, and five flavors on the functions of five *zang*-organs, six fu-organs, five constituents, and five sense organs. For example, the liver (wood) corresponds with wind in spring in the east; the heart (fire) corresponds with heat in summer in the south; the spleen (earth) corresponds with dampness in late summer in the central region; lungs (metal) correspond with dryness in autumn in the west; kidneys (water) correspond with cold in winter in the north. Therefore, only when the human body corresponds with the external environmental variations and seasonal changes, can the harmonious man-nature relation be maintained.

The application of Five Elements in physiology can be generalized into the following three points. First, based on the properties of Five Elements, five *zang*-organs, along with their related five constituents, five sense organs, and five emotions, etc., form a physiological unity and manifest the holism of the human body. Second, abiding by interpromotion and interrestraint, five *zang*-organ systems mutually promote and restrain to form an organic integrity. Third, the human body and nature are correspondent for their attributes of Five Elements.

However, the theory of Five Elements is not perfect in explaining medical problems. First, it is not comprehensive enough to expound all the attributes of five *zang*-organs with Five Elements. For example, Five Elements can explain one of the functions of the liver(wood), namely the liver governing *shu xie* (dredging the routes and regulating the movement of *qi*) in that it prefers freedom to stagnation, accordant with the wood's attributes of flexing, extending, and developing; however, it fails to expound its another function, i.e., the liver storing blood, because wood has no property of storage.

The second limitation of Five Elements is that interrestriction and interpromotion of Five Elements fail to expound all the interrelationships between organs. Among Five Elements, water restraining fire corresponds with kidneys restraining the heart. However, it neglects the fact that kidneys and the heart can promote each other, which is called "coordination between water and fire" by the ancient Chinese. In terms of interpromotion, metal promoting water is used to elucidate the relation between the lungs and kidneys, i.e., with the lungs as the upper source of water, lung-*qi* descends to make water return to and nourish the kidneys. But it is hard to explain why the essence in kidneys can nourish the lungs.

The above illustrations show that we should avoid the mechanical application of the theory of Five Elements in understanding the intrinsic functions of viscera, tissues, and organs, as well as their internal relationships.

5.3.5.2 Explanation of Etiology and Pathogenesis

According to the theory of Five Elements, human physiology corresponds with outside climate, five tastes, and inner emotions.

First, abnormal climates can affect man's physiological functions and cause diseases. *Plain Questions*, Chapter 5 states that the excess of wind, heat, dampness, dryness, and cold will impair the corresponding viscera. Excess wind in spring impairs the liver, excess heat in summer hurts the heart, excess dampness in late summer damages the spleen, excess dryness in autumn impairs lungs, and excess cold in winter impairs the kidneys.

Second, excessive emotional changes (anger, joy, contemplation, grief, and fear) will directly damage the corresponding visceral functions, leading to the emotional diseases. For instance, anger is controlled by the liver, but rage impairs the liver; joy is governed by the heart, while ecstasy harms the heart; contemplation is controlled by the spleen, while excessive contemplation does damage to the spleen; grief is dominated by the lungs, but excessive grief impairs the lungs; fear is dominated by the kidneys, while excessive fear injures the kidneys.

Third, the flavors in a daily diet may also be responsible for some diseases. *Plain Questions*, Chapter 3 shows that five flavors of foods nourish five *zang*-organs respectively, but if excessively taken, they will impair five *zang*-organs. Excessive sour impairs the liver; excessive bitter harms the heart; excessive sweet damages the spleen; and excessive acridness injures the lungs; excessive saltiness hurts the kidneys.

Exogenous pathogenic factors, excessive emotional changes, and excessive flavors always impair the corresponding viscera. It is the so-called "pathogenic factors impairing the corresponding viscera in Five Elements." However, the theory is not a mechanical formula in pathology. Other specific conditions like "excessive five flavors all can impair the spleen and stomach" should be taken into due consideration.

5.3.5.3 Explanation of the Transmission and Prognosis of Diseases

Five *zang*-organs are interrelated in physiology and mutually influential in pathology. Diseases of various *zang*-organs may mutually transmit, which is called "transmission." There are three ways of transmission: interpromotion transmission, interrestraint transmission, and temporal transmission.

- **Interpromotion Transmission**

It involves two transmitting directions: mother-child transmission and child-mother transmission, namely "the disorder of the mother organ involving the child organ" and "the child organ affecting the mother organ."

"The disorder of the mother organ involving the child organ" means that a disease is transmitted from the mother organ into the child organ, such as the liver disease transmitting into the heart, the heart disease into the spleen, the spleen disease into the lungs, the lung disease into the kidneys, and the kidney disease into the liver. Clinically, the insufficiency of the mother organ results in the insufficiency of the child organ, and finally results in the deficiency of both the mother organ and the child organ. A typical example is "the insufficient essence and blood of the liver and kidneys." Normally, the mother organ, kidneys (water), can promote its child organ, the liver (wood). However when the mother organ is not abundant enough to promote its child organ, i.e., "water fails to moisten wood," the child organ will become weaker.

"The disorder of the child organ affecting the mother organ" means that a disease is transmitted from the child organ into the mother organ, such as liver disease transmitting into the kidneys, kidney disease into the lungs, lung disease into the spleen, spleen disease into the heart, and heart disease into the liver. Clinically, it ends up with the disorder of both child organ and mother organ. It covers two aspects. The first is "the disease of the child organ involving its mother organ." Namely, excess syndrome of the child organ leads to the excess syndrome of both the child organ and mother organ by involving the mother organ. For example, the hyperactivity of heart-fire may bring on the hyperactivity of liver-fire, resulting in the superabundance of both heart-fire and liver-fire. The second aspect is "the child organ consuming *qi* of the mother organ." Namely, the deficiency of the mother organ results from the insufficiency of the child organ. For instance, the spleen (earth) is the child of the heart (fire). In physiology, the spleen absorbs food nutrients and transforms them into blood, for the heart guarantees the normal blood circulation. In pathology, the dysfunction of the spleen results in the deficiency of both the spleen and heart, and causes the disorder of the heart. Anther example is that since the lungs are the mother of kidneys, the function of lungs governing respiration ensures that the kidneys absorb enough qi, which is called "lungs are the governor of qi and kidneys are the root of qi." But the deficiency of kidney-qi leads to the failure of the lungs to disperse and descend, bringing on the disorder of both the lungs and kidneys with the symptoms of dyspnea and shortness of breath.

- **Transformation of Interrestraint**

The transformation of interrestraint covers overrestraint and counterrestraint.

Overrestraint refers to the transmission of a disease due to excessive restraint, the order of which is the same as that of interrestraint, i.e., liver disease transmitting into the spleen, spleen disease into the kidneys, kidney disease into the heart, heart disease into the lungs, and lung disease into the liver. There are two causes for overrestraint transmission. One is that one element among Five Elements becomes too powerful and thus overrestrains the one which it is normally superior to; the other possible reason is that one element becomes too weak and therefore it is overrestrained by the one which it is normally inferior to. A good case in point is the relationship between the liver and the spleen. An excessively powerful liver will overrestrain the spleen and stomach, which is called "wood over-restraining earth;" excessively weak spleen will be excessively restrained by the liver, which is termed as "deficient earth being over-restrained by wood."

Clinically, "wood overrestraining earth" means that the excessive *shu xie* (dredging and regulating) of liver-qi will affect the digestion of the spleen and stomach. To be specific, the excessive *shu xie* of liver-qi can cause dizziness, headache, irritability, anger, chest oppression, and hypochondriac pain; if liver disease is transmitted into the spleen, symptoms of spleen asthenia such as abdominal distension, abdominal pain, anorexia, loose stool, and retention of feces will appear; if the stomach is involved, it will manifest as anorexia, belching, acid regurgitation, and vomiting, which are the symptoms of stomach-qi dysfunction. When pathogenic factors transmit from the dominator into the submitter, diseases are relatively severe, for the lately affected organ was overrestrained by the originally affected organ.

Unlike overrestraint, counterrestraint refers to the transmission of a disease due to opposite restraint, the order of which is just contrary to interrestraint, namely liver disease into the lungs, lung disease into the heart, heart disease into kidneys, kidney disease into the spleen, spleen disease into the liver. There are also two reasons for counterrestraint transmission. One is that one element among Five Elements becomes too powerful and thus counterrestrains the one that it is normally inferior to; the other is that one element becomes too weak and therefore it is counterrestrained by the one that it is normally superior to.

Take the liver's counterrestraining the lungs for example. The exuberance of liver-fire leads to the disorder of the lungs in depuration and descent. The manifestations concerning the liver are pains in the chest and hypochondria, bitter taste in the mouth, irritability and susceptibility to anger, as well as taut and rapid pulse; and the manifestations concerning the lungs are cough with sputum or even hemoptysis. When pathogenic factors transmit from the submitter to the dominator, as Xu Dachun pointed out, diseases are relatively mild, for the lately affected organ restrains the originally affected organ in physiology.

From the above descriptions, we can see that the disease of any *zang*-organ can be transmitted from and into the other four *zang*-organs through "the disorder of the mother organ involving the child organ," "the disorder of the child organ affecting the mother organ." Take the liver for example. Both "liver disease transmitting into the heart" and "kidney disease transmitting into the liver" pertain to "the disorder of mother organ involving the child organ"; both "liver disease transmitting into kidneys" and "heart disease transmitting into the liver" pertain to "the disorder of the child organ affecting the mother organ"; both "lung disease transmitting into the liver" and "liver disease transmitting into the spleen" pertain to overrestraint transmission; both "spleen disease transmitting into the liver" and "liver disease transmitting into lungs" pertain to counterrestraint transmission (Figure 5-21).

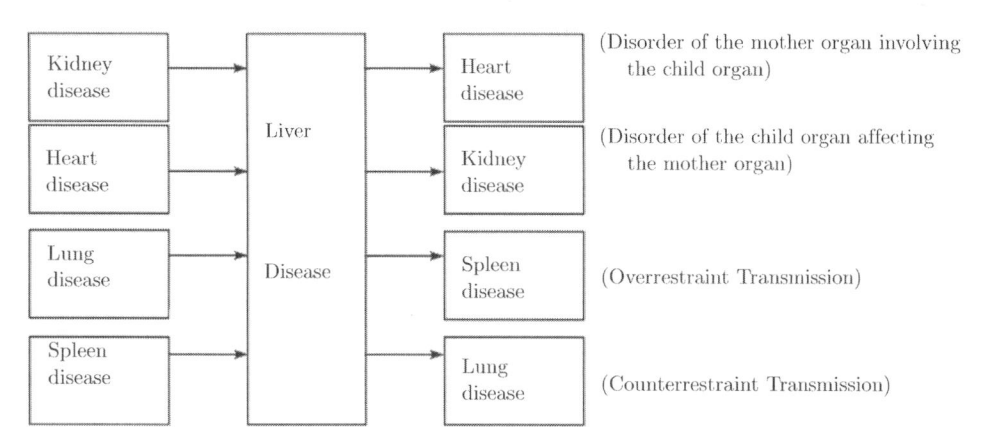

Figure 5-21 Transmission among Diseases of Five *Zang*-organs

- **Temporal Transmission of Diseases**

For one thing, different seasons and climates exert different influences on diseases, which can also be explained with the theory of Five Elements. Five seasons and five *zang*-organs correspond with each other for the same attributes of Five Elements. Spring and the liver pertain to wood, summer and the heart to fire, late summer and the spleen to earth, autumn and lungs to metal, and winter and kidneys to water. Therefore, seasonal changes may directly lead to the occurrence, development, and prognosis of diseases. *Plain Questions*, Chapter 22 says that "liver disease has to be cured in summer, otherwise it will get worse in autumn, extend into winter, and relapse in the next spring." Specifically, since summer (fire) is the child of the liver (wood), liver disease turns to the help of the child to be recovered; since autumn (metal) is the dominator of the liver (wood), liver disease gets worse out of being restrained by its dominator, and even extends into winter and relapses the next spring (wood) which is governed by the liver.

For another, for the different attributes, day and night have a different influence on diseases. Dawn pertains to wood, noon to fire, afternoon to earth, dusk to metal, and night to water. Diseases of five *zang*-organs are mild at its dominant time, severe at the time which its dominator governs, and relatively mild at the time that its mother governs. According to *Plain Questions*, Chapter 22, "heart disease is mild at noon, for it is the heart's dominate time; it is severe at night, for it is time when the heart's dominator governs; and it is relatively mild at dawn, for it is the mother of the heart who governs."

5.3.5.4 Guiding Clinical Diagnosis

The human body is an organic integrity. In terms of their attributes of Five Elements, five *zang*-organs, along with their related *fu*-organs, constituents, sense organs, emotions, colors, notes, flavors and *qi*, form five interpromoting and interrestraining physiological systems, with five *zang*-organs at the centers. The disorders of the internal organs can manifest themselves through outer tissues. Therefore, the pathological changes of the internal organs can be inspected through the observation of the external complexion and luster, voice, as well as posture and pulse condition. Through the long-term accumulation of clinical experiences, the ancient Chinese have created four diagnosis methods: inspection, auscultation and olfaction, interrogation, and pulse taking and palpation.

- **Inspection**

Physicians diagnose diseases and syndromes by observing the patients' constituents, sense organs, colors, etc. Specifically, to obtain information for a diagnosis, physicians should observe the patient's mental state, facial expression, complexion, physical conditions, skin color, tongue and coating, as well as the changes of urine, stool, and other excreta. Pathological features such as the spasm and convulsion of muscles and four limbs, upward staring of eyes, and bluish complexion are the general indicates of liver disease. The reason is that the liver pertains to wood, governs tendons, opens into the eyes, and corresponds with green in colors. According to TCM, the facial color and luster are the sighs of visceral essence. *Plain Questions*, Chapter 17 points out that the normal facial color with luster shows sound function of the viscera. In addition, the complexion can reflect the type of disease, e.g., both bluish and blackish complexion indicate pain syndrome, both yellowish and reddish complexion indicate heat syndrome, and whitish color indicates cold syndrome.

- **Auscultation and Olfaction**

Five sounds, five notes, and five smells correspond with five *zang*-organs respectively, so physicians can deduce the affected *zang*-organ from the abnormal changes in sound, note, and smell. For instance, the incoherent speech, constant curse, and uncertain mood are the indications of mania due to the disorder of heart-spirit. The symptoms of cough, asthma, low and weak voice, and fishy sputum usually are the indications of lung disease.

- **Interrogation**

Physicians can deduce the affected *zang*-organ by inquiring of patients about the etiology, the season of onset, the abnormal taste in the mouth, and emotional changes. For example, the liver tends to be attacked by a pathogenic wind in spring, and the spleen tends to be affected by dampness in late summer; bitter taste in the mouth is the manifestation of the exuberance of heart-fire, and sweet taste in the mouth indicates spleen disease; excessive grief tends to impair the lungs, and excessive fear tends to damage the kidneys.

- **Pulse Taking and Palpation**

Pulse conditions vary with seasons, for five *zang*-organs correspond with five seasons. Under normal conditions, as the liver, spring and taut pulse all pertain to wood in Five Elements, the slightly taut pulse in spring is the indication of the favorable condition of the liver; as the heart, summer and full pulse all pertain to fire, the full pulse in summer indicates the health of the heart; as the spleen, late summer and slow pulse all pertain to earth, the slightly slow pulse in late summer shows the soundness of the spleen; as the lungs, autumn and floating pulse all pertain to metal, the floating pulse in autumn manifests the strength of the lungs; as the kidneys, winter and deep pulse all pertain to water, the slightly deep pulse in winter reflects the normality of the kidneys.

Through inspection, auscultation and olfaction, interrogation, and pulse taking and palpation, physicians acquire some clinical symptoms and physical signs, categorize them in terms of the attributes of Five Elements, and then decide the diagnosis. The liver disease can be diagnosed by the symptoms pertaining to wood such as bluish complexion, a preference for sour flavor, hypochondriac pain, dizziness, susceptibility to rage, and taut pulse. Heart disease is characterized by the symptoms pertaining to fire like reddish complexion, bitter taste in the mouth, irritability, and full pulse. The spleen disease is manifested with the symptoms pertaining to earth such as yellowish complexion, sweet taste in the mouth, vomiting, diarrhea and bloating, as well as thin pulse. The lung disease is represented by the symptoms pertaining to metal such as whitish complexion, cough, stuffy nose, susceptibility to sadness, and floating pulse. And the kidney disease is indicated by the symptoms pertaining to water such as blackish complexion, salty taste in the mouth, seminal emission, impotence, enuresis, weakness of the waist and knees, susceptibility to fear, and deep pulse.

5.3.5.5 Guiding Clinical Treatment

Guided by the theory of Five Elements, physicians can control disease transmission and decide effective therapeutic principles and methods.

- **Controlling Disease Transmission**

Under certain conditions, diseases of one *zang*-organ can transmit into other *zang*-organs, according to the laws of interpromotion, interrestraint, overrestraint, and counterrestraint of Five Elements. Specifically, excess syndrome of one *zang*-organ can transmit into its submitter organ via overrestraint, into its dominator via counterrestraint, and even into its mother organ. One *zang*-organ with deficiency syndrome can be affected by its dominator via overrestraint or by its submitter via counterrestraint, and at the same time, its disorder can also transmit into its child organ via interpromotion. The mastery of the transmission laws enables physicians to cut down the transmission, and control the disease where it breaks out. However, one point has to be borne in mind, i.e., physicians should select the viscera subject to transmission for treatment. For example, liver disease, according to the theory of Five Elements, tends to transmit to the heart, lungs, spleen, and kidneys. However, clinically the organ that is more frequently to be affected by the liver disease is the spleen, so preventive measures should be taken in advance to protect the spleen in the treatment of the liver disease.

- **Deciding Therapeutic Principles and Methods**

Usually the therapeutic principles and methods are decided according to the laws of interpromotion and interrestraint. They can be summarized as follows.

Principle 1: To decide therapeutic methods according to the law of interpromotion: to reinforce the mother organ and purge the child organ.
    Maxim 1: To reinforce the mother organ
        Method 1: To enrich water to nourish wood
        Method 2: To supplement fire to reinforce earth
        Method 3: To enrich earth to generate metal
        Method 4: Mutual promotion between metal and water
    Maxim 2: To purge the child organ
        Method 1: To purge the heart to treat the excess syndrome of the liver
        Method 2: To purge the spleen to treat the excess syndrome of the heart
        Method 3: To purge the kidney to treat the excess syndrome of lungs
Principle 2: To decide therapeutic methods according to the law of interrestraint: to inhibit the strong and support the weak.
    Maxim 1: To inhibit the strong, supplemented by supporting the weak
    Maxim 2: To support the weak, supplemented by inhibiting the strong
        Method 1: To inhibit wood and support earth
        Method 2: To reinforce metal to inhibit wood
        Method 3: To purge fire and supplement water

To Decide Therapeutic Methods according to the Law of Interpromotion

It is also known as "to reinforce the mother organ" and "to purge the child organ," for respectively "the disorder of the mother organ involves the child organ," and "the disorder of the child organ involves the mother organ."

The first therapeutic maxim, "to reinforce the mother organ," is used to treat the deficiency syndrome of both mother organ and child organ. For example, the deficiency syndrome of liver-*yin* and kidney-*yin* due to the failure of insufficient kidney-*yin* to nourish liver-*yin* should be treated by reinforcing kidney-*yin*, for kidneys (water) can promote its child organ, the liver (wood). Another example is that the deficiency syndrome of both spleen-*qi* and lung-*qi* caused by the insufficiency of lung-*qi* should be treated by reinforcing spleen-*qi* for the spleen (earth) can promote its child organ, lungs (metal).

The followings are the essential therapeutic methods to reinforce the mother organ.

"To enrich water to nourish wood" is applicable to the deficiency syndrome of liver-*yin* due to the insufficiency of kidney-*yin*. The method is to nourish liver-*yin* by reinforcing kidney-*yin*, and therefore it is also known as "nourishing kidney to strengthen the liver."

"To supplement fire to reinforce earth" is applicable to the deficiency syndrome of kidney-*yang* caused by the insufficiency of spleen-*yang*. This method is used to supplement spleen-*yang* by reinforcing kidney-*yang*, and therefore is also named "to reinforce kidneys to strengthen the spleen." It should be noticed that according to interpromotion among Five Elements, the heart pertains to fire, the spleen pertains to earth, and thus "fire failing to promote earth" means that the heart fails to promote the spleen. However, since the theory of *life gate* was put forward in the Ming dynasty, "fire failing to promote earth" usually refers to the deficiency syndrome of both spleen-*yang* and kidney-*yang* due to the insufficiency of kidney-*yang* (the fire of *life gate*).

"To enrich earth to generate metal" is a method used to supplement lung-*qi* by reinforcing spleen-*qi*, which is also called "to supplement the spleen to strengthen lungs." It is applicable to the deficiency syndrome of spleen-*qi* and lung-*qi* due to spleen-*qi* insufficiency.

"Mutual promotion between metal and water" is a method used to treat the deficiency syndrome of lung-*yin* and kidney-*yin* by supplementing lung-*yin*, also known as "to supplement lungs to nourish kidneys." It is applied to treating the deficiency syndrome of kidney-*yin* caused by failing of deficient lung-*yin* to nourish the kidneys and the deficiency syndrome of both lung-*yin* and kidney-*yin* due to the failure of deficient kidney-*yin* to nourish the lungs.

The second therapeutic maxim is "to purge the child organ." It is applicable to the excess syndrome of both mother organ and child organ, or the excess syndrome of the mother organ. For instance, the excess syndrome of the liver due to the hyperactivity of liver-fire or the excess syndrome of the heart and the liver caused by the hyperactivity of heart-fire can be treated by purging heart-fire because the heart is the child organ of the liver. The main therapeutic methods of purging the child organ include "to purge the heart to treat the excess syndrome of the liver," "to purge the spleen to treat the excess syndrome of the heart," and "to purge kidneys to treat the excess syndrome of lungs."

To Decide Therapeutic Methods according to the Law of Interrestraint

This therapeutic principle is also known as "to inhibit the strong and support the weak." The abnormal state of interrestraint includes overrestraint and counterrestraint. The organ overrestraining or counterrestraining other organs is called strong, otherwise it is weak. Inhibiting the strong and supporting the weak should be used in combination together, though they have different weights concerning different syndromes.

"To inhibit the strong, supplemented by supporting the weak" is a therapeutic maxim applied to overrestraint and counterrestraint. For example, the adverse flow of liver-*qi* tends to invade the spleen, and brings on its dysfunction, which is called "wood overrestraining earth." And thus it should be treated by inhibiting wood, supplemented by supporting earth (also known as inhibiting the liver and strengthening the spleen). On the contrary, if the obstruction of spleen-*qi* affects the function of the liver, viz. earth counterrestrains wood, it should be treated by inhibiting earth, supplemented by supporting wood (also termed as inhibiting the spleen and strengthening the liver).

"To support the weak, supplemented by inhibiting the strong" is another therapeutic maxim applied to the deficient interrestraint. For instance, if kidney-*yin* fails to nourish heart-*yin* due to its own insufficiency, it will lead to heart-*yang* hyperactivity, which is called "water failing to restrain fire," and should be treated by supporting kidney-*yin*, supplemented by inhibiting heart-*yang*.

The followings are the essential therapeutic methods decided according to the law of interrestraint.

"To inhibit wood and support earth" is a method used to treat the syndrome of liver hyperactivity and spleen weakness by inhibiting the liver and strengthening the spleen. It is applicable to the syndrome of wood's overrestraining earth.

"To reinforce metal to inhibit wood" is a method used to treat the disorder of lungs in depuration and descent due to liver-fire superabundance. Specifically, physicians try to inhibit the liver and help lung-*qi* depurate and descend.

"To purge fire and supplement water" is a method used to treat the excess syndrome of heart-*yang* due to kidney-*yin* insufficiency by supplementing kidney-*yin* and purging heart-*yang*, which is also known as "nourishing *yin* and purging fire."

Guiding Acupoint Selection

In acupuncture and moxibustion, the five-*shu* acupoints, which are located on the distal extremities of hands and feet, respectively pertain to Five Elements, that is, Jing-Well acupoint pertains to wood, Ying-Spring acupoint to fire, Shu-Stream acupoint to earth, Jing-River acupoint to metal, and He-Sea acupoint to water. In the treatment of visceral diseases by acupuncture and moxibustion, acupoints are selected according to the nature of diseases. *Classic of Medical Problems: Liu Shi Jiu Nan* insists on "reinforcing the mother in treating deficiency syndrome and purging the child in treating excess syndrome."

As to deficiency syndrome, the technique of "reinforcing the mother" is applied by acupuncturing the mother-acupoint on its own meridian or the acupoints pertaining to the same element as the mother-acupoint on its mother meridian. For example, for the deficiency syndrome of the liver (wood), its mother organ is water, and thus it should be treated with reinforcing technique by acupuncturing the LR8-water-acupoint (He-Sea acupoint) on the liver meridian of foot *jueyin*, or acupuncturing the KI10-water-acupoint (He-Sea acupoint) on its mother meridian, the kidney meridian of foot *shaoyin*.

As to excess syndrome, the technique of "purging the child" is applied by acupuncturing the child-acupoint on its own meridian or the acupoint pertaining to the same element as the child-acupoint on its mother meridian. For example, for the excess syndrome of the liver (wood), the child of the liver is fire, and therefore it should be treated by reducing technique, specifically acupuncturing the LR2-fire-acupoint (Ying-Spring acupoint) on the liver meridian of foot *jueyin*, or acupuncturing the HE8-fire-acupoint (Ying-Spring acupoint) on its child meridian, the heart meridian of hand *shaoyin*.

- **Guiding Psychotherapy**

Psychotherapy is mainly used to treat emotional diseases. Five kinds of emotions interrelate with five *zang*-organs, and thus interpromotion and interrestraint also exist among five emotions. Since emotions restrain each other in physiology and are closely related to internal organs in pathology, interrestraint among emotions can be applied to treating emotional diseases. *Plain Questions*, Chapter 5 states that "excessive rage impairs the liver, and grief restrains rage; excessive joy impairs the heart, and fear restrains joy; excessive contemplation damages the spleen, and rage restrains contemplation; excessive grief damages lungs, and joy restrains grief; excessive fear impairs kidneys, and contemplation restrains fear." The reasons are as follows.

As to the emotion of lungs, grief pertains to metal; as to the emotion of the liver, rage pertains to wood. Metal can restrain wood, so grief restrains rage. As to the emotion of kidneys, fear pertains to water; as to the emotion of the heart, joy pertains to fire. Since water can restrain fire, fear restrains joy. As to the emotion of the liver, rage pertains to wood; as to the emotion of the spleen, contemplation pertains to earth. Since wood can restrain earth, rage restrains contemplation. As to the emotion of the heart, joy pertains to fire; as to the emotion of lungs, grief pertains to metal. Fire can restrain metal, and therefore joy restrains grief. As to the emotion of the spleen, contemplation pertains to earth; as to the emotion of kidneys, fear pertains to water. Since earth can restrain water, contemplation restrains fear.

- **Guiding Clinical Medicine and Nutritional Medicine**

Medicine and the a diet of various flavors respectively nourish various *zang*-organs and the constituents of human body. For example, sour nourishes the liver and bitter nourishes the heart. Medicine and a diet fail to nourish a certain *zang*-organ due to the fact that the insufficiency of a certain flavor causes the deficiency of this *zang*-organ; on the contrary, medicine and a diet with a certain excess flavor will impair a certain *zang*-organ. Therefore, the former should be treated by nourishing this *zang*-organ with the medicine or a diet with the flavor of the same element; the latter should be treated by purging the excess flavor with the flavor of its dominator. For example, the insufficient spleen-*qi* should be supplemented with the medicine or a diet sweet in flavor, for sweet flavor (earth) can nourish the spleen (earth); if the medicine or a diet of excessive sour impairs the liver, it should be treated by purging sour with the medicine pungent in flavor, for pungent flavor (metal) can restrain sour flavor (wood).

Besides, a diet with various flavors can also help the body recover. For instance, patients with dampness in the spleen or diabetes should take no or less sweet food; patients with edema due to kidney-*yang* insufficiency should take no or less salty food; patients with liver-*yin* deficiency should take sour food.

The laws of interpromotion and interrestraint are of practical values in treatment. However, not all mental diseases can be treated with the theory of Five Elements. Such a theory will be more effective when used with other theories together.

5.4 Interrelationships among Theories of Primordial *Qi*, *Yin-yang*, and Five Elements

These three theories are all ancient philosophical thoughts imbued with materialism and dialectics. They have promoted the establishment and the development of TCM's theoretical system and are of great values in clinical practice, and therefore have become the essential components of TCM. As a natural view, the theory of primordial *qi* lays the theoretical fundament for TCM; as methodology, the theories of *yin-yang* and Five Elements establish the basic framework for TCM's theoretical system.

Yin-yang theory and the theory of Five Elements are based on the theory of primordial *qi*. They all regard *qi* as the original foundation of the universe. They all hold that a system itself has the potential of self-regulating and maintaining a dynamic equilibrium. These similarities enable them to cooperate in expounding complex physiological activities, studying complicated pathological changes, and effectively guiding specific clinical practices.

CHAPTER 6

Model, Method, and Architecture of TCM

Objectives & Requirements
1. Development of medical models and the main contents of a new medical model.
2. Peculiar connotation of TCM's model.
3. General philosophical methods of TCM.
4. Specific practical methods of TCM.
5. TCM's architecture and curriculum.

Key Concepts
1. A medical model is the general understanding of medical thought including ethical spirit, medical theory and practice, as well as its development. As an ancient medical system, TCM has its distinctive ethical concept and medical theory; the formation and development of its medical model embody unique characteristics and rich scientific contents.
2. TCM not only has its unique philosophical methodology, it has created varied empirical methods to guide its practice.
3. TCM's architecture consists of various interrelated parts, covering various basic and clinical subjects, as well as theories and methods of health maintenance.

6.1 The Model of TCM

Medicine is an exploration of life phenomena, as well as disease prevention and treatment. At the same time, it is a process where people develop practical experiences into scientific theory, which in turn further guides practice. In this process, through educational and academic activities, people standardize their understandings and form medical models. A medical model includes medical thinking, ethical spirit, medical developmental strategy, and all medical techniques. Thus, it is a kind of theoretical generalization about all medical phenomena. The birth and evolution of a medical model always correspond with the level of human knowledge. The world's medical models have developed from primitive psychic-medical model, to natural-philosophical-medical model, to mechanical-medical model, then to biological-medical model, and finally to the modern bio-psycho-social-medical model.

6.1.1 Preliminary Establishment of The Bio-psycho-social-medical Model

People have tried to establish various medical models. The earliest one is the psychic-medical model, which believes in the doctrine of God. Due to the lack of scientific knowledge, ancient people were not able to provide reasonable explanations for many natural phenomena, so they attributed those unexplainable things to the deeds of supernatural powers. They held that God dominated everything, even the health of human beings; diseases were the punishments from God. Therefore, they turned to witchcraft to expel the devil or prayed to God to forgive them.

Human cognition about man, nature, and disease improves with the development of technology, economy, and society. the psychic-medical model was challenged. People began to search for the origin of diseases from the aspects of natural philosophy, and then natural-philosophical-medical model came into being. In China, along with the philosophical doctrine of *yin* and *yang* formed 2,000 years ago, the pathological concepts of *qi* and blood, as well as Five Elements appeared around A.D. 300, have shed light on the essence of disease and treatment. Such a model is of great historical and realistic significance.

The Renaissance in Italy has promoted the progress of science and technology, especially in celestial mechanics and mechanical mechanics. The materialist philosophy revived and developed in the form of mechanism. Meanwhile, humanism also rose with the slogan: "we are human beings; we are entitled to know everything about ourselves." This historical background gave rise to the mechanical-medical model, which believed that all the movement in nature, including man's, is a mechanical one. Rene Descartes' book *Animals Are Machine* and Julien Offray de La Mettrie's work *Man Is Machine* are the representatives of such kinds of thought. In their books, it is claimed that disease is the malfunction of some part of a machine, and the doctor is the technician. Under the influence of this kind of mechanical-medical model, medical science underwent a revolutionary progress in anatomy, histology, and so on. Andreas Vesalius's remarkable contribution in anatomy and Rudolf Virchow's pathology of the cell all laid a solid foundation for the development of modern medicine. However, mechanics have neglected both the biological characteristics of human life and the social complexity, so it inevitably leads to one-sidedness and superficiality.

The widespread application of microscopes propelled the development of biological science by leaps and bounds. With the discovery of a series of microorganism's pathogenesis at the end of the 19th century, the biomedical viewpoint turned out to be the mainstream of medical thought, consequently forming the biological-medical model. It studies disease and health about their cause, host, and environment. The model has played a positive role in modern medicine. A case in point is that the three primary inventions in the first half of this century, i.e., prophylactic inoculation, sterilization, and disinsectization, as well as antibiotics, have drastically lowered the rate of incidence and the mortality of acute and chronic diseases as well as parasitic diseases in a few dozens of years alone. However, its starting point was pure biology; it merely emphasized the biological factors of diseases. When it comes to the host of the disease, it merely took physiology and pathology into consideration; as far as environment is concerned, it just focused on the change of natural environment. With the development of society and the progress in medicine itself, its inherent shortcoming of one-sidedness turned increasingly obvious, especially when chronic illness became one main threat to man's health.

As social modernization is speeding up, man's living conditions, behavior patterns, and even psychological activities have changed a lot. Therefore, cardiovascular diseases, malignant tumors, and the accident injuries have taken a lead in the disease and death spectrums. For one thing, the main threatening diseases have gradually transformed from infectious diseases into noncommunicable ones, and therefore the former bio-medical model appears helpless. For another, in underdeveloped and developing countries, infant mortality is still very high, and communicable diseases are still the most serious medical problem.

In the modernized society, the ever-tensing working pressure, heated competition, and quick-life rhythm make people more likely to get mental diseases. The American Academy of Family Physicians (AAFP) estimates that 60% of patients suffer psychological stress, which results in harmful lifestyles, such as excessive drinking, smoking, excessive eating, and negative emotions, and thus lead to tumors and coronary artery disease.

At the same time, as a social undertaking, medical science becomes more and more important. People begin to realize that health service does not merely belong to medical institutions, but is a public undertaking. In the West, the universal repugnance against those bad behaviors like taking drugs and excessive drinking has urged governments to take social measures, and in some countries, healthcare policy and environmental pollution control even become important issues in presidential campaigns. The United Nations and the World Health Organization (WHO) call for all governments to bring health service into the state's economic and social development plan, and take health as a social investment.

The modernization and civilization of social life make people have a new understanding of health. To be healthy is to stay in a normal state in both psychology and society. A man's biological attribute and social attribute require doctors and even the entire health service system to appraise both people's morbid and normal states.

In 1974, A. Friede and H.L. Blum first proposed an environmental-health-medical model, i.e., environmental factors, and particularly social factors have great influence on people's health. In order to clarify the disease causes and expound the impact of diseases on health, Marc Lalonde and G. E. Alan Dever set forth the overall-health-medical model based on health policy analysis. Later in 1977, an international psychiatry conference was held in Canada. Many scholars attach great importance to mental disease prevention through social measures. The patient's social attributes should be taken into account in diagnosis. G.L.Engel, the professor of psychiatry and medicine in the University of Manchester put forward the bio-psycho-social-medical model after the conference. This new model soon attracted the world's attention and won identification in the medical field.

The bio-psycho-social-medical model accords with the concept of health proposed by WHO. Being healthy is not only a state free from disease and infirmity, but also a state of physical, mental, and social health. Being unhealthy is no longer a biological notion, concerning discomforts or pain deformities, but the constraints in work, study, and response capacity. The main points of the bio-psycho-social-medical model can be stated in the following five aspects. (a) Man is a social entity, whose health is mainly decided by the social factors; (b) to be healthy is to be psychologically and socially sound enough; (c) medical science is of the nature of social and natural sciences; (d) a doctor is not a medical biologist alone and he is a medical psychologist and medical socialist as well; (e) the task of a health service is not to relieve patients of diseases alone, and it is also to reform humans in psychology and society; (f) getting rid of diseases to safeguard health depends on the improvement of social and natural conditions.

The progress from the bio-medical model to the bio-psycho-social model is not only a great theoretical leap, but also has a significant effect on the healthcare practice, for it requires that doctors have a full understanding of disease causes by evaluating the patient's psychological state and social background.

In terms of health service, the impacts of the bio-psycho-social medical model are as follows. Medical practice has expanded (a) from treatment to prevention services; (b) from physical to psychological services; (c) from hospital services to outside services; and (d) from technical services to social services. As to the management of health undertaking, the modern medical model provides the best analyzing and decision-making model. A case in point is that any plan for healthcare facilities, and the organization and working system of a health service must combine prevention and treatment together.

As far as medical education is concerned, the bio-psycho-social-medical model promotes the medical education from the traditional isolated way into a modern one. Some humanities and interdisciplinary-sciences are added into the curriculum, such as psychology, sociology, ethics, social medicine, philosophy of medicine, and health economics. Teaching also puts emphasis on the combination of theory and practice, arming future doctors with both a higher professional quality and better professional ethics.

The new medical model suits a community's requirement for high-quality health services. The understandings of health and disease become increasingly comprehensive, covering prevention, rehabilitation, and treatment. Many medical achievements have been made with the new medical model. A good case in point is that the mortality of cardiovascular disease has declined sharply.

6.1.2 TCM's Peculiar Model and Its Principle

Taking in the latest achievements of world medicine, Chinese people apply the new bio-psycho-society-medical model in its traditional medicine background, and form its unique medical model, that is, the environment-body-mind medical model.

This model has two theoretical cornerstones. The first one is that man is the unity of the body and mind. Namely, it is an organic entity of both physical and mental attributes. In the TCM model, the body refers to man's physical structures such as viscera, meridians-collaterals, muscles, and life substances like *qi*, blood, and body fluids; the mind is a psychological notion, covering various psychological activities such as feeling, thinking, and desiring. The body and mind are dialectically related, i.e., the body is the premise of the generation of mental activities, physical activities are influenced by mental states, and the unity of the body and mind ensures the human life.

The second cornerstone of the TCM model is that man's body and mind, as well as their activities, are influenced by their natural and social conditions. *The Classic of Internal Medicine* holds that "man correlates with the heaven and the earth, and corresponds with the shift of the sun and the moon," i.e., man's functional activities are affected by natural conditions. In addition, social conditions such as political, economical, and cultural factors, as well as individual social status, relations, and experiences all affect man's body and mind.

On these two cornerstones, the TCM model establishes its peculiar principle: any medical practice, including diagnosis, treatment, prevention and healthcare, is to take man's physical and mental conditions, as well as various environmental factors, into consideration. Such a principle runs through the whole theoretical system of TCM.

In etiology, the principle of the TCM model is manifested as the theory of "three etiologic factors," namely, endogenous factors, exogenous factors, and others. Exogenous factors mainly refer to those natural conditions that affect man's physiological functions; and endogenous factors and others cover such aspects as society, psychology, and individual behaviors (emotional change, improper diet, overwork, and overrest, etc.).

In diagnosis, the principle is abided by in four diagnostic methods (inspection, auscultation and olfaction, interrogation, and pulse taking and palpation) and the process of syndrome differentiation. According to *The Classic of Internal Medicine*, a good doctor is to inquire about four seasonal and geographical features of the place the patient live in, interpersonal relationships, living conditions and social status, as well as the patient's individual characteristics, such as dietary habits and character traits.

In therapy, the principle functions as a guideline. For one thing, TCM emphasizes that treatment should adapt to such natural conditions as season and geography. For instance, an astringent should not be applied in spring and summer, for *yang-qi* was exuberant in these two seasons, and an astringent would lead to fever due to *yang-qi* stasis; a dispersing agent should not be used in autumn and winter, for *yang-qi* was weak in these two seasons, and a dispersing agent would cause cold syndrome due to dissipation of *yang-qi*. Similarly, cold medicines like *Gypsum Fibrosum* (gypsum) should be avoided in winter, and hot medicines like *Radix Aconiti Lateralis Preparata* (root of common monkshood) should be avoided in summer.

For another, in treatment, doctors should also consider such social conditions as a patient's economic condition, political position, cultural cultivation, local customs, experiences, living habits, and dietary habits. The therapeutic experiences of "four great physicians in Jin and Yuan Dynasties" are typical cases. Li Gao, the father of the "spleen-invigorating" school, was born in wars and learned that a person's spleen and stomach were likely to be hurt by his drifting life, and therefore presented the essential clinical treatment, "to warm and invigorate spleen and stomach"; Zhang Congzheng, the initiator of "purgation" school, advocated that pathogenic factors should be driven out by means of diaphoresis, emesis, and purgation, for people at that time preferred a tonic and thus many excess syndromes appeared; Zhu Zhenheng, the founder of "nourishing *yin*" school, born in the Yangtze River region, usually used the therapeutic method of nourishing *yin* to reduce fire in treatment, because he realized that people in that area are *yin*-asthenia-featured and usually took pungent and dry herbs that are likely to generate interior fire; Liu Wansu born in North China, the founder of "the school of cold and a cool," believed that "fire and heat" were the main causes of diseases and therefore should be treated with medicines of cold and a cool nature, because he found that North China was dry with insufficient rain and people preferred meat, and thus many heat syndromes appeared.

Besides, as to the psychological factors, ancient Chinese created many psychotherapies like verbal comforting and persuading, emotional diversion, and medicinal regulation. The model and its principle also require that doctors try to stimulate healthy psychological activities in patients to establish a cooperative relation between doctors and patients.

The fourth manifestation of the principle of the environment-body-mind-medical model is in medical prevention. First of all, people are to obey the objective laws of environmental changes to form a good habit of health cultivation; second, people should properly deal with their social and individual vicissitudes to establish a correct life philosophy; finally people are to maintain a sound mental condition to prevent diseases.

To sum up, the basic principle of the TCM model runs through the whole theoretical system of TCM and plays a leading role in its diagnosis, treatment, and medical prevention. During more than 2,000 years, medical scientists in various dynasties have been unceasingly enriching and developing the TCM system through the long-term practice and finally make the TCM model more perfect. The rich medical practice and reasonable connotation of the TCM model have provided references and enlightenment for the development of contemporary medicine.

6.2 The Method of TCM

Method is the sum of the means by which people either acquire empirical facts of scientific theory, or establish theoretical system with empirical facts. TCM's general philosophical methods explain the essence of life; and its specific research methods guide the practical medical activities.

6.2.1 General Philosophical Methods of TCM

TCM's general philosophical methods are its holistic approach, system approach, and dialectical approach, corresponding with TCM's philosophical concepts of holism, Five Elements, and *yin-yang*.

The holistic approach has three connotations. First, nature and man are united as a whole. The man-nature correspondence decides the likelihood of analogy between them. Namely, we can understand human physiological and pathological changes by observing the corresponding natural phenomena. For example, the physiological function of lung depuration can be understood from the analogy: Lungs pertain to metal in Five Elements, and therefore like metal, they have the natures of depuration, astringency, and descent. Second, the exterior and interior of the human body are related in a unity, and thus the cognitive method of "speculating the interior from the exterior" is generated. For example, TCM holds that the heart-blood condition mainly displays itself on the face, therefore the observation of complexion and luster enable us to understand the condition of the heart and blood. The ruddy and lustrous face shows the sufficiency of the heart blood. With this method, *zang-xiang* theory is established. Third, the unique diagnostic methods of TCM (inspection, auscultation and olfaction, interrogation, and pulse taking and palpation) also result from the holistic approach. In terms of the holistic approach, the local is included and reflects the whole, and therefore such diagnostic methods as tongue examination, complexion examination, pulse examination, and abdomen examination are to analyze and judge the whole state of the patients.

The second approach, system approach, attaches importance to the classification and connection of interrelated elements which constitute comparatively stable systems. In TCM, the system method is mainly reflected in the theory of Five Elements, which holds that all things in nature can be classified into five categories according to their attributes, i.e., wood, fire, earth, metal, and water. They are interpromoting and interrestraining. Such a system method enables people to understand the internal order and organic connection of the human body, and requires people to deal with medical problems starting from the cognition of the complicated relationship. Take the *zang-xiang* theory as an example. Besides the cognition of physiological functions and characteristics of various *zang-fu* organs, in terms of the theory of Five Elements, we must understand the role of every *zang* and *fu* organ in the whole life system and its connection with other organs. Another case is for syndrome differentiation in clinical practice, according to the theory of Five Elements, we should understand not only the essential features and clinical manifestations of different syndromes, but also their internal connection, mutual influence, and transformation.

The last approach, a dialectical approach, is a means by which people cognize things dialectically with the concept of "unity of opposites." It is fully reflected in the *yin-yang* theory which maintains that everything is a contradictory unity of *yin* and *yang*. Let's take human respiratory function, for example. Expiration (*yang*) and inspiration (*yin*) are opposite but interdependent. There will be no inspiration without expiration and vice versa. In one breath, expiration is the process of *yang* waxing and *yin* waning, and inspiration is the opposite. Expiration turns into inspiration when it reaches its peak, and vice versa. The conversions from expiration to inspiration and that from inspiration to expiration form a respiratory cycle, whose relative equilibrium is achieved by their wane-wax and transformation.

Among general philosophical approaches, the holistic approach promotes people to understand human health and disease from a macroscopic perspective; the system approach explores the intrinsic relationships of various systems in the human body; and the dialectical approach guides ancient doctors to establish various levels of TCM theory.

6.2.2 Specific Research Methods of TCM

Guided by the fundamental philosophical methods, i.e., holistic, dialectical and system approaches, ancient Chinese have created many distinguishing specific research methods to guide medical observation, experiment, and theoretical reflection.

6.2.2.1 Making an Analogy

The method of analogy is a logical reasoning used to infer some characters of an unknown object from those of a familiar one based on the assumption that two things alike in some aspects are similar in others. In ancient China, analogy has become one of medical research methods, as *Plain Questions,* Chapter 76: *Diagnose According to he Established Norm in a Leisured Way* says, experienced doctors investigate both the human body and diseases by analogy based on previous knowledge in astronomy, geography, and sociology. First, to explain the physiological functions of the internal organs, *Plain Questions,* Chapter 8: *The Confidential Collections in the Royal Library about the Functions of the Twelve Viscera* make such an analogy between the official ranks in the feudal society and various organs: "as the monarch of the human body, heart dominates human spirit, ideology and thought; like an officer who is in charge of the granary, the spleen takes charge of the digestion and absorption of foods; like an officer who takes charge of water, the urinary bladder is responsible for storing and discharging urine." Second, to analyze human pathology, *The Classic of Internal Medicine* compares human blood to rivers. A river congeals into ice at a low temperature and thaws at a high temperature. Analogically, the blood stream stagnates when the human body is attacked by pathogenic cold, and turns smooth when treated with warming therapy. In addition, the method of analogy is also applied in treatment. For instance, the therapeutic method "increasing body fluids to relieve constipation" is created by the analogy of natural phenomenon that a boat can be steered in rivers with the buoyancy of water. Similarly, constipation due to *yin*-deficiency caused by the insufficiency of body fluids should be treated by nourishing *yin* to induce defecation.

The method of analogy is feasible in understanding human physiology, pathology and treatment based on the cognition of the natural world. However, an analogy is a logical reasoning from one particularity to another particularity, so the theory deduced from it is of a great probability and thus is to be validated in practice.

6.2.2.2 Speculating the Interior from the Exterior

This method is an ancient cognitive method. *Spiritual Pivot,* Chapter 75: *The Criterions of Pricking and the Difference Between Healthy Energy and the Evil Energy* points out that we can judge the size and quality of a piece of wetland from the condition of the reeds on it. Similarly, the close relationship between exterior manifestations of the human body and its interior changes determines that we can understand the physiological and pathological changes of the interior organs from their exterior manifestations.

With this research method, ancient Chinese established the *zang-xiang* theory. Wang Bing in the Tang Dynasty explained that "*xiang* is the exterior manifestations of things or phenomena." And Zhang Jiebin in the Ming Dynasty gave a clearer statement: "*xiang* means visible appearance, manifesting the *zang-fu* organs residing in the human body, so the correspondence is called *zang-xiang* (*Classified Canon*)."

6.2.2.3 Heuristic Method

The heuristic method refers to a research method by which a hypothesis is proved. However, its purpose is not confined to proposing and verifying a hypothesis, but is to understand the nature and reveal the truth. The heuristic method is widely applied in TCM and lots of theories are thus created. For example, *The Classic of Internal Medicine* puts forward the theory of a man-nature correspondence. Ancient Chinese hold that the fullness of the moon has an influence on human physiology and pathology. Just as *Spiritual Pivot,* Chapter 79: *On the Dews of the Year* states, "When full moon occurs, human *qi* and blood is sufficient, and the muscular interstices are dense. When the moon disappears on the first day and the last day of the lunar month, human *qi* and blood is insufficient, and the muscular interstices are loose, and thus if attacked by pathogenic wind, diseases are much likely to occur." In addition, TCM holds that the alternation of day and night also has an impact on the progression of diseases to a certain extent. *Spiritual Pivot,* Chapter 44: *The Human Healthy Energy in the Day and Night Corresponds with the Energies of the Four Seasons* states that "most of diseases turn light at dawn and keep stable in the daytime, aggravate in the evening and get even worse at night," because "at dawn, *yang-qi* of the human body begins to form and pathogenic factors decline, during the daytime *yang-qi* grows and defeats the pathogenic factors; in the evening, *yang-qi* starts to decline and pathogenic factors begins to generate; at night, *yang-qi* is stored into the viscera and pathogenic factors reside alone in the body." It shows that the conditions of a disease varies with the changes of *yang-qi* in the day, corresponding with the alternation of day and night. This explanation is obviously a hypothesis, which has been used for over two thousand years by TCM. Until modern time, with the study of chronobiology and chronomedicine on biological clock phenomena, the rationality of the theory has not been proved and developed.

The heuristic method is applied widely in the clinical practice of TCM. Different diseases may have similar symptoms, which makes it hard to make a precise diagnosis on some critical but complex diseases in a short time. Doctors have to make an impression diagnosis and give temporary but emergent treatment based on their own knowledge and experiences. Guided by the heuristic method, doctors have to observe diseases further, revising diagnosis and improving treatment based on the therapeutic effect and the change of the disease state, until the finial diagnosis is made. *Treatise on Febrile Diseases* states that "if a patient has not defecated for about a week, there may be dry feces in his large intestine. Doctors can cautiously try *Xiao Chengqi Tang*. If the patient farts after taking this prescription, it proves that dry feces really exist in the large intestine, and then purgative method can be used." The similar illustrations are numerous in ancient medical books.

One thing is worth noting. Safety is the prerequisite to the heuristic method, either in the theoretical research or in testing a new therapeutic medicine, technology, or method. Deliberate measures, skillful techniques, and attentive operations are the requirements of this method.

6.2.2.4 Counterevidence

It is a kind of indirect reasoning, namely speculating one thing with the aid of its reverse side, for some natures are much easier to be observed in an abnormal state. Accordingly, TCM often appeals to the sharp contrast between the normal and abnormal conditions of viscera to inspect the physiological functions, pathological changes, and the nature of etiology.

TCM counterproves their physiological functions of the internal organs from the pathological manifestations. For example, through long-term observation, ancient Chinese found that the disorder of lungs could lead to such symptoms as adverse rising of lung-*qi*, dyspnea, cough and expectoration, and spleen disease can be manifested as abdominal distension, diarrhea, lassitude of limbs, weakness, and even edema. Based on these pathological manifestations, ancient doctors acquired the cognition that lungs have the functions of dominating respiration and governing depuration and descent, and the spleen functions in transforming food and water, as well as transporting body fluids. Take six *fu*-organs for another example. Gastric disorder may be manifested as nausea, vomiting, and eructation, and intestinal diseases caused by constipation may be manifested as abdominal distension, abdominal pains and vomiting, and thus ancient doctors found that the smooth transmission was the normal functional state of six *fu*-organs, i.e., six *fu*-organs work well when they were not obstructed. Another example is that ancient doctors found that patients with exuberance of liver-fire always had such symptoms as redness, swelling, and pain of the eyes, and patients with liver-*yin* insufficiency always had blurred vision and even night blindness. Based on these pathological manifestations, ancient medical experts drew the conclusion that the liver opened into the eyes.

Through this method, TCM also deduces pathogenesis from the physiological functions of internal organs. For instance, since lungs govern depuration and descent, cough and dyspnea are always caused by the lungs' failure to depurate and descend; the liver opens into the eyes, so reddish and swollen eyes are usually caused by the exuberance of liver-fire. The counterevidence between reason and result is based on the massive clinical data and long-term clinical practice. This method plays a very important role in the studies of physiology, pathology, cause of disease, diagnostic method, syndrome differentiation, treatment, medicine, and so on.

6.2.2.5 The Method of Insight

The sudden realization of the essence of things after long deliberation is called "insight." It is the sudden enlightenment based on previous knowledge and experiences. As a unique cognitive method in TCM, it refers to the sudden realization of the essence of the human body and diseases based on previous medical knowledge or experiences. It is widely applied in the clinical practice of TCM. With this method, ancient medical experts created many medical classics such as *Clinical Experiences of Zhu Danxi*[84] and *Insight from Medical Study*.[85] Based on his own therapeutic experiences and the related theory that "all the epidemic diseases are infectious, with similar symptoms"(*Plain Questions*), Wu Youke (a famous physician in the Ming dynasty) got the sudden insight that the cause of an epidemic disease is a kind of special evil *qi* rather than such abnormal climatic factors as wind, cold, summer-heat, dampness, dryness and heat. He composed the *Treatise on Pestilence* to elaborate epidemic-disease transmission, the law of occurrence, and the therapeutic methods. Wu Tang (an expert in the Qing dynasty) wrote in the preface to his work *Wenbing Tiao Bian*[86] that "Through the long-term clinical practice and learning of medical theories, I have been constantly pondering various medical problems and finally have some new understandings and apperceptions about medical theories, and hereby compose the book." Similarly, Cheng Guopeng in the Qing dynasty carefully studied various therapeutic methods and relationship between them, and then generalized the therapeutic methods into eight categories: diaphoresis, emesis, purgation, regulating therapy, warming therapy, cooling therapy, supplementing, and resolving therapies. All of the above are the cases of insight in points.

As a kind of creative thinking, the method of insight plays an important role in scientific research. However, it has such limitation as subjectivity, and thus the theory obtained with this method needs further proving.

6.3 The Architecture of TCM

The TCM system is an organic whole composed of interrelated knowledge. It is composed of two subsystems: the theoretical system and the clinical system. To wind the whole introduction to TCM, here is a general summary of these two essential components, which have been expounded in Chapter 2, Chapter 3, Chapter 4, and Chapter 5.

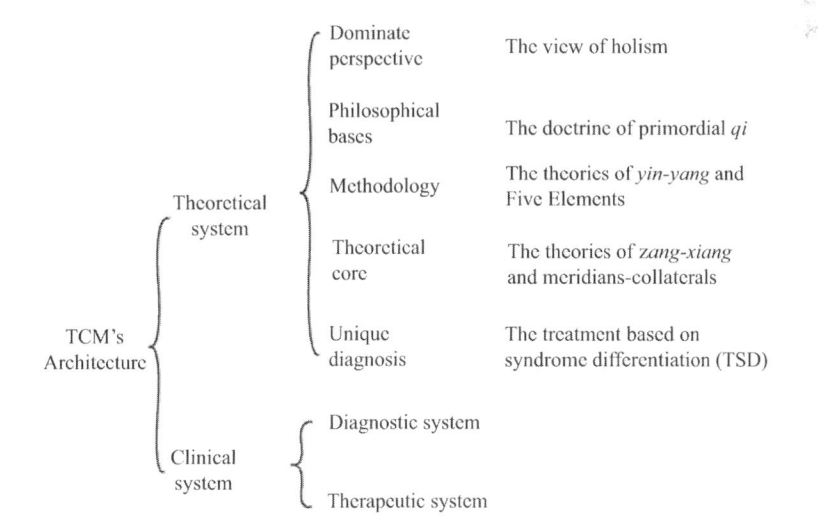

TCM's Architecture
- Theoretical system
  - Dominate perspective: The view of holism
  - Philosophical bases: The doctrine of primordial *qi*
  - Methodology: The theories of *yin-yang* and Five Elements
  - Theoretical core: The theories of *zang-xiang* and meridians-collaterals
  - Unique diagnosis: The treatment based on syndrome differentiation (TSD)
- Clinical system
  - Diagnostic system
  - Therapeutic system

6.3.1 A Summary of the Fundamental Theories of TCM

The fundamental theories of TCM are the bases for its development. Its formation is based on thousands of years' medical practice and theoretical reflection, influenced by ancient Chinese cultures especially by its natural philosophical thoughts. They have absorbed the contemporary scientific achievements and investigated the relationship between man, nature and disease.

The theoretical system takes holism as its fundamental perspective, the doctrine of primordial *qi* as its philosophical guideline, the theories of *yin-yang* and Five Elements as its methodology, the theories of *zang-xiang* and meridians-collaterals as its theoretical core, and the principle of treatment based on syndrome differentiation (TSD) as its main diagnostic feature.

The view of holism, as the dominant perspective of TCM, lays stress on the unity between man and nature, the unity between body and mind, and the integrity of the human body itself. It attributes disease to the imbalance of the holistic relation of the human body, and thus any treatment should center on the overall adjustment of the human body.

The doctrine of primordial *qi* provides an important philosophical basis for TCM to understand the essence of nature, human life, and disease. The human body results from the accumulation of *qi*; human functional activities depend on the promotion of *qi*; and human psychological phenomena such as feeling, thinking, and emotion are the results of *qi* activities. The abnormal movement of *qi* causes various pathological factors, and therefore the focus of treatment is to regulate and restore *qi* balance.

Yin-yang and Five Elements are philosophical concepts of ancient China. They explain the generation and the change of the nature with the contradictory unity of *yin-yang*, and they also expound the complex interrelationship with the principles of interpromotion and interrestraint among Five Elements. In the process of its formation and development, TCM, with the theories of *yin-yang* and Five Elements, establishes such medical theories as body-mind unity, *zang-fu* organs and meridians-collaterals, pathogenesis, and therapeutic principles.

Zang-xiang and meridians-collaterals are the cores of TCM theory. Based on the concept of holism, the theories of *zang-xiang* and meridians-collaterals first elucidate human life activities, physiological functions, and pathological changes with the method of "speculating the interior from the exterior," and then study the human *zang-xiang*, body, spirit, meridians-collaterals, *qi* and blood with the views of "holism," "constant movement," and "universal relation."

TSD, a unique method to analyze, study, and treat diseases under the guidance of holism, is the basic principle of disease identification and treatment, and is one of the basic features of TCM. TSD requires that doctors determine the proper therapies according to time, individuality, and geographical environment; it emphasizes "focusing on the principal cause of disease"; it maintains that the ultimate objective of syndrome differentiation is to differentiate between *yin* and *yang*; finally it puts forward that the ultimate goal of treatment is to maintain the *yin-yang* balance.

Note: Major Courses about TCM's Fundamental Theories

- **A General Introduction to Traditional Chinese Medicine**

It is an introductory course that mainly covers the property, nature, medical model, and method of TCM; it also studies the history, present situation, and development of TCM. The objective of the course is that learners have a general view of the architecture and characteristics of the theoretical system of TCM, as well as some basic viewpoints of TCM theory.

- **Science of *Zang-xiang* of Traditional Chinese Medicine**

It is a basic course about human physiology, in which the theories of *zang-xiang* and meridians-collaterals are the core of the theoretical system of TCM. The theories of *qi*, bloods and body fluids combined with the theories of *zang-xiang* and meridians-collaterals form the peculiar physiological cognition of TCM. The theory of constitution focuses on human physiological characteristic and relevant medical problems.

- **Science of Etiology and Pathogenesis of Traditional Chinese Medicine**

It is a basic discipline about the disease cause and pathological knowledge, including three major parts: (a) etiology that analyzes various pathogenic factors and their pathogenic features; (b) the science of pathogenesis that discusses the intrinsic mechanism and general law of diseases' development and evolution; (c) the science of the onset of diseases that elaborates the mechanism of the occurrence of disease and dialectical relation between endogenous pathogenic factors and exogenous factors.

- **Diagnostics of Traditional Chinese Medicine**

It is a bridge between the basic disciplines and the clinical disciplines in TCM. It mainly introduces four diagnostic methods of TCM (namely inspection, auscultation and olfaction, interrogation, and pulse taking and palpation), the objective and modern study progress of four diagnostic methods, as well as the basic training of four diagnostic skills.

- **Science of Syndrome Differentiation of Traditional Chinese Medicine**

It is a basic discipline that expounds the theoretical principles, methods, and skills of syndrome differentiation, and introduces the common clinical syndromes and the key points of syndrome differentiation. It deepens and synthesizes the theoretical cognition of *zang-xiang* etiology and pathogenesis of TCM. The mastery of this discipline will be helpful in both understanding related fundamental theories and making correct syndrome differentiation in clinical practice.

- **Schools of Traditional Chinese Medicine**

It aims at improving learners' theoretical level of TCM. It introduces the unique opinions of famous medical experts in the past dynasties, their contributions to the fundamental theories of TCM, and their important clinical practice. Through this course, learners are expected to broaden their medical vision.

- **The History of Traditional Chinese Medicine**

It is a course about the historical process and the law of TCM development. With a historical and scientific approach, the course is expected to arm its learners with a clear understanding of the past, the present, and the future of Traditional Chinese Medicine.

- **Science of Chinese *Materia Medica***

It introduces the theoretical knowledge of Chinese Materia Medica as well as the nature, characteristics, indication, and efficacy of common medicinal herbs. All of them are the bases of other courses for Science of Chinese *Materia Medica* and Science of Prescriptions.

- **Science of Prescriptions**

It is the bridge between the basic disciplines and the clinical disciplines of TCM. It introduces the principles of prescription composition and the related theoretical knowledge of prescription. The course also selectively introduces the composition, main efficacy and modification of some representative prescriptions.

6.3.2 A Summary of the Clinical System

The clinical system of TCM is gradually formed based on fundamental theories and therapeutic technology. It involves specific cognition of various diseases as well as their therapeutic measures, methods, and experiences. Its therapeutic and diagnostic systems are the reflection of the view of holism and TSD of TCM.

Note: Major Courses about the Clinical Discipline of TCM

- **Internal Medicine of Traditional Chinese Medicine**

As a main course of the clinical discipline of TCM, it mainly introduces the relevant medical theories, as well as the diagnosis and treatment of common diseases of internal medicine.

- **Surgery of Traditional Chinese Medicine**

As a main course of the clinical discipline of TCM, it mainly introduces the relevant medical theories, the diagnosis and treatment of common surgical diseases, as well as the common surgical manipulation and techniques. It can be divided into such branches as dermatology of TCM, enterology of TCM, and the science of acute abdominal diseases of TCM.

- **Traumatology and Orthopedics of Traditional Chinese Medicine**

It is a unique clinical course that introduces the relevant medical theories, the diagnosis and treatment of common diseases in traumatology and orthopedics, as well as their common manipulation and techniques.

- **Gynecology and Obstetrics of Traditional Chinese Medicine**

It is a unique clinical course that introduces the relevant medical theories, and the diagnosis and treatment of common gynecologic and obstetrical diseases.

- **Pediatrics of Traditional Chinese Medicine**

It introduces the physiological and pathological characteristics of infants and children, the relevant medical theories, as well as the diagnosis and treatment of common pediatric diseases, and pediatric skills.

- **Ophthalmology of Traditional Chinese Medicine**

It introduces the anatomical structure of the eyes, and expounds TCM's cognitions of the physiology and pathology of the eyes. It also investigates the relation between the eyes and viscera, the relevant medical theories, the diagnosis and treatment of common ophthalmologic diseases, and some operational skills of TCM ophthalmology.

- **Otorhinolaryngology of Traditional Chinese Medicine**

It introduces the anatomical structures of the ears, nose, pharynx and larynx, and expounds TCM's cognitions of their physiology and pathology. It also studies the relations between the ears, nose, pharynx, larynx and viscera, the relevant medical theories, the diagnosis and treatment of common diseases, and some operational skills.

- **Science of Acupuncture and Moxibustion of Traditional Chinese Medicine**

As a main course of the clinical discipline of TCM, it mainly introduces the relevant medical theories, and the indication and operational skills of acupuncture and moxibustion. It can be divided into such branches as the science of meridians and collaterals; the science of acupoints, experimental acupuncture and moxibustion; the therapeutics of acupuncture and moxibustion; the science of healthcare through acupuncture and moxibustion; the philology of acupuncture and moxibustion; as well as various schools' theories of acupuncture and moxibustion.

- **Massage Science of Traditional Chinese Medicine**

It introduces the relevant medical theories, the indication and operational skills of massage, with healthcare through massage as one focus.

- **Classics Reading 1:** *Treatise on Febrile Diseases*

The course is designed to improve learners' clinical skills and enrich their clinical knowledge by introducing Zhang Zhongjing's therapeutic experiences of exogenous diseases.

- **Classics Reading 2:** *Synopsis of Golden Chamber*

The course is designed to improve learners' level of TSD concerning internal injuries by introducing Zhang Zhongjing's therapeutic experiences of internal injuries.

Main References

He Yumin. 1987. *An Introduction to Traditional Chinese Medicine*. Shanghai: Shanghai College of Traditional Chinese Medicine Press.

Jia Dedao. 1993. *A General History of Traditional Chinese Medicine*. Taiyuan: Shanxi Science and Technology Publishing House.

Li Dexin. 1994. *Basic Theories of Traditional Chinese Medicine*. Changsha: Hunan Science and Technology Publishing House.

Li Guohao, Zhang Mengwen, and Cao Tianqing. 1986. *The History of Chinese Science and Technology*. Shanghai: Publishing House of Shanghai Ancient Books.

Liu Wushun, Xiao Xishou, Yang Tingqi, and Jiao Chunrong. 1994. *Enlightenment from Contemporary Medicine Development*. Beijing: Publishing House of Chinese Medicine Science and Technology.

Qiu Peiran and Ding Guangdi. 1992. *Various Theories of TCM*. Beijing: People's Health Publishing House.

Wu Tunxu. 1995. *Fundamental Theories of Tradition Chinese Medicine*. Shanghai: Shanghai Science and Technology Publishing House.

Xie Zhufan. 2002. *Classified Dictionary of Traditional Chinese Medicine* (New Edition). Beijing: Foreign Languages Press.

Xue Yu. 1984. *Chinese Pharmaceutical Historical Data*. Beijing: People's Health Publishing House.

Yan Shiyun. 1989. *Chinese Academic History*. Shanghai: Shanghai College of Traditional Chinese Medicine Press.

Yin Huihe. 1984. *Fundamental Theories of Tradition Chinese Medicine*. Shanghai: Shanghai Science and Technology Publishing House.

Yu Shenchu. 1987. *Historical Outline of Chinese Materia Medica*. Kunming: Yunnan Science and Technology Publishing House.

Yuan Yixiang, Ren Jixue, and Huang Long (eds.). 1996. *Chinese-English Dictionary of Traditional Chinese Medicine*. Beijing: The People's Medical Publishing House.

Zhang Zhenyu. 1993. *Basics of Traditional Chinese Medicine*. Beijing: Traditional Chinese Medicine Press.

Zhang Zhenyu. 1988. *An Introduction to Traditional Chinese Medicine*. Jinan: Shangdong College of Traditional Chinese Medicine Press.

Zhou Yimou. 1983. *The Ages of Medical Ethics*. Changsha: Hunan Science and Technology Publishing House.

Zhou Yimou and Xiao Zuotao. 1988. *A Collection of Selected Medical Books in Mawangdui*. Tianjin: Tianjin Science and Technology Publishing House.

Fan Qiaoling. 2002. *Science of Prescriptions*. Shanghai: Publishing House of Shanghai University of Traditional Chinese Medicine.

Zhang Youjun, Li Zhi, and Zheng Min. 1995. *Chinese-English Chinese Traditional Medical Word-Ocean Dictionary*. Taiyuan: Shanxi People Publishing House.

Harriet Beinfield and Efrem Korngold. 1992. *Between Heaven and Earth: A Guide to Chinese Medicine*. New York: Ballantine Books.

O'Shaughnessy Michelle D.O.M. 2008. *Traditional Chinese Medicine*. Carol Stream, Illinois: Allured Pub. Corp.

Endnotes

[1] Shennong, together with Suiren and Fuxi, was called "Three Emperors" by the Chinese. It was said that Shennong was the founder of agriculture and traditional Chinese medicine.

[2] *Huainan Tzu* (*Huainan Zi*) was complied by Huainan prince Liu An (in the Western Han dynasty, 202 B.C.–8 A.D.) and his hanger-ons Li Shang, Su Fei, Wu Bei, etc. The book is a representative of Taoism-legalist combination, expounding such essential philosophical doctrines as Taoist *Yin-yang*, Confucianism and Mohism.

[3] *Plain Questions* (*Su Wen*) is one of the two parts of *The Classic of Internal Medicine*, dealing with a variety of subjects, such as man's anatomy, physiology, etiology, pathology, diagnosis, etc. The book emphasizes the idea of holism in TCM's theoretical construction. Its theories about y*in-yang*, Five Elements, *zang-xiang*, and meridians are important theoretical sources of TCM.

[4] *The Classic of Internal Medicine* (*Huangdi Nei Jing* or *Nei Jing*) is one of the four greatest medical classics extant in China, with its authorship ascribed to the ancient Emperor Huangdi (2698–2589 B.C.). Actually the work was a product of various unknown authors in the Warring States Period (475–221 B.C.). Its core content is Emperor Huangdi's questions to Qi Bo (a medical physician) about the occurrence, development, and treatment of diseases. The whole book is divided into two parts: *Spiritual Pivot* (or *The Classic of Acupuncture*) and *Plain Questions*.

[5] *History of the Later Han Dynasty* (*Han Shu*) is the first chronological dynastic history of China edited chiefly by Ban Gu in the Eastern Han dynasty (25–220 A.D.), covering the history from 202 B.C. to 23 A.D.

[6] *Records of the Historian* (*Shi Ji*) is the first biographical history in China. It was written by Sima Qian in the Han dynasty (206 B.C.–220 A.D.). It covers the biographical sketches of emperors, feudal lords, and important historical events.

[7] *The Book of Songs* (*Shi Jing*) is the earliest anthology of poems in China, complied in Zhou dynasty (1046–256 B.C.). More than 300 poems accounts for the 500 years of Chinese social life.

[8] *The Classic of Mountains and Rivers* (*Shan Hai Jing*) was complied in the pre-Qin period. It covers ancient legends, geography, products, witchery, religion, history and medicine, etc. It is composed of 18 volumes; and more than 100 states, 550 mountains, and 300 rivers are described.

[9] *Treatise on Exogenous Febrile Diseases and Miscellaneous Diseases* (*Shanghan Zabeing Lun*) is one of the four greatest medical classics extant in China. It was accomplished by Zhang Zhongjing at the beginning of the 3rd century. Diagnosis and treatment of fevers and other miscellaneous diseases are dealt with in the book. It is composed of the *Treatise on Febrile Diseases* (mostly concerning exogenous febrile diseases) and the *Synopsis of the Golden Chamber* (concerning more about the internal damages and their treatment). Clinically, most herbal formulae from the book are really effective and still extensively used by herbalist doctors till now, such as *Mahuang Tang* (Ephedra Decoction), *Guizhi Tang* (Decoction of Cassia Twig), *Xiao Qinglong Tang* (Minor Green Dragon Decoction), *Wumei Wan* (Black Plum Pill), etc.

[10] *The Classic of Medical Problems* (*Nan Jing*) appeared in the 1st or the 2nd century B.C., authorship unknown. It is one of the theoretical classics of TCM. It is believed that the book was finished before the East Han dynasty (25–220 A.D.). In the form of questions

and answers, the book deals with such medical aspects as the acupoints for acupuncture and moxibustion, the methods of needling, the physiological and pathological conditions related to the meridians and collaterals, and the methods of pulse-taking.

[11] *The Classic of Materia Medica (Shennong Ben Cao Jing)* is China's earliest *materia medica*, believed to be a product in the 1st century B.C., with its authorship attributed to the ancient emperor Shennong. In the book 365 kinds of drugs are listed and divided into three classes: superior, common, and inferior.

[12] *The General Treatise on the Etiology and Symptomatology of Diseases (Zhu Bing Yuan Hou Lun)*, as its name suggests, is the earliest treatise on etiology and symptomatology of various diseases, with its focus on internal medicine. It was finished in about 610 by doctors such as Chao Yuanfang. As a summarization of the previous achievements of TCM, it collected, classified, and compiled various clinical experiences.

[13] *Therapeusis of Pediatric Diseases (Xiaoer Yao Zheng Zhi Jue)* was compiled by the famous doctor Qian Yi in the Song dynasty (960–1279 A.D.). It mainly investigates the physiology, pathology, diagnosis, and treatment of pediatric diseases. Besides pediatric diseases, it has tackled other medical issues.

[14] *Prescriptions Assigned to the Three Categories of Pathogenic Factors of Diseases (San Yin Ji Yi Bing Zheng Fang Lun)*, compiled in 1174 by Chen Yan, was generally acknowledged as the greatest podiatrist in Chinese medicine. It classifies the causes of disease into external, internal, and miscellaneous ones which are regarded as neither external nor internal.

[15] *Corrections of the Errors in Medical Works (Yilin Gaicuo)* was compiled in 1830 by Wang Qingren, who insisted on making anatomical observations and had made studies of dozens of years on the internal organs of the human body. In this book the author corrected certain mistakes made by past generations concerning the internal organs, and suggested new methods of treating blood stasis and hemiplegia. His method of promoting the blood and removing stasis is still of practical value.

[16] *The Pulse Classic (Mai Jing)*, written by Wang Shuhe in the 3rd century, is generally acknowledged as the standard work on the pulse conditions, channel terminologies, and pulse methods, etc.

[17] *The Classic of Acupuncture (Zhen Jing)* is one essential part of *The Classic of Internal Medicine*, focusing on the meridian treatment with needles.

[18] *Acumoxibustion on Mingtang Acupoint (Mingtang Kong Xue Zhenjiu Zhi Yao)* was the earliest book on acupuncture in China with the authorship unknown in the Qin and Han dynasties (221 B.C.–220 A.D.).

[19] *The A-B Classic of Acumoxibustion (Huangdi San Bu Zhenjiu Jia Yi Jing)* is composed by physician Huangpu Mi (215–282) in about 256–259. It is one of the classic of acumoxibustion based on *Plain Questions*, *The Classic of Acupuncture* and *Acumoxibustion on Mingtang Acupoint*.

[20] *A Handbook of Prescriptions for Emergencies (Zhou Hou Beiji Fang)* is believed to be originally compiled by Ge Hong (283–343, a Taoist scholar and physician), in which the prescriptions recorded are simple and the drugs used are common and effective, and many valuable descriptions of diseases and treatments are recorded.

[21] *Medical Secrets of an Official (Wai Tai Mi Yao)*, compiled in 752 by Wang Tao is a comprehensive summary about TCM's achievements before the Tang dynasty (618–907 A.D.). It is composed of 40 volumes about exogenous diseases, internal medicines, etc., with 1,104 issues of medical problems discussed and over 6,000 prescriptions recorded.

[22] *The Taoist Lin's Secret Recipes for Wounds and Bone-setting (Lin Daoren Xian Shou Li Shang Xu Duan Mifang)* was the earliest monograph on traumatology extant in China. It was accomplished by an orthopedics physician in the Tang dynasty (618–907 A.D.), whose surname name is Lin, but first name is still unclear, and therefore he was called Taoist Lin

(about 790–850) because of his religion.

[23] *Effective Prescriptions Handed Down for Generations* (*Shi Yi De Xiao Fang*) (1345) was composed by the Yuan dynasty's physician Wei Yinlin, on the basis of the author's family experiences as physicians for five successive generations. There are nineteen volumes in all, covering thirteen medical branches such as internal medicine, surgery, gynecology, and pediatrics. But its main achievements are in orthopedics and traumatology.

[24] *Prescriptions for Midwifery* (*Bei Chan Ji Yong Fang*) was written by Yu Liu in 1140. Just as its name suggests, the book provides many effective recipes to midwifery.

[25] *Treatise on Infant Health and Pediatric Prescriptions* (*Xiaoer Weisheng Zong Wei Fang Lun*) (1156) is a classic on pediatrics by an anonymous physician. It is a comprehensive summary of pediatrics before the South Song dynasty.

[26] *Well-tried Formulas by Su and Shen* (*Su Shen Liangfang*) is believed to be compiled in the Song dynasty by an anonymous researcher according to *Su's Recipes* by Su Shi (1037-1101, the famous litterateur and calligrapher of the Northern Song dynasty), and statesman of the Song dynasty) and *Well-tried Formulas* by Shen Kuo (1031–1095, a polymathic Chinese scientist and statesman of the Northern Song dynasty). The book is composed of ten volumes, covering pulse, *zang-fu* theory, herbs and moxibustion, etc.; it also sheds light on otolaryngology, surgery, internal medicine, etc. It is photocopied by the People's Public Health Publishing Company in 1956.

[27] *The Classified Materia Medica* (*Zheng Lei Ben Cao*), was composed by Tang Shenwei at the end of the 11th century. It lists 1,746 kinds of medicine with directions for use and preparation.

[28] *Six Legal Documents of Tang Dynasty* (*Tang Liu Dian*) was composed by Zhang Shui, Zhang Jiuling, and annotated by Li Linfu (one of the prime ministers in the Tang dynasty) and others. The book was finished in 738, and is the earliest book on China's political and legal system.

[29] *The Compendium of Materia Medica* (*Ben Cao Gang Mu*) (1596) was compiled by Li Shizhen, who spent 30 years on 52 volumes. It lists 1,892 medical substances, more than 1,000 illustrations and over 10,000 prescriptions with detailed descriptions of the appearance, properties, methods of collection, as well as preparation and use of each substance. The book is far more than a pharmaceutical compendium; it is also a comprehensive work on various branches of natural science, including botany, zoology, mineralogy, and metallurgy.

[30] *Treatise on Pestilence* (*Wenyi Lun*) was composed by Wu Youke in 1642. It embodies two volumes. There are 50 chapters in the first volume, and 36 in the second. The first volume accounts for the cause, pathogenesis, and treatment of pestilence, and the second volume focuses on the concomitant syndromes of pestilence.

[31] *Chiseling Open the Regularity of Qian (Heaven)* (*Qian Zao Du*) is an important philosophical monograph on "changes" in the Han dynasty (206 B.C.–220 A.D.).

[32] *Spiritual Pivot* (*Ling Shu*) is one essential part of *The Classic of Internal Medicine*, and focuses on meridian treatment with needles.

[33] *Synopsis of the Golden Chamber* (*Jinkui Yao Lue*) is one essential part of *Treatise on Exogenous Febrile Disease and Miscellaneous Disease*. It focuses on the internal damages and their treatment. There are 25 Chapters with 262 herbal formulae.

[34] *Zuo Commentary* (*Zuo Zhuan*) is the earliest and the first complete chronicle historical records in China. It is believed to be composed by Zuo Qiuming (556–451 B.C.) to expound ON Confucius's work *Spring and Autumn* (*The History of Lu State*). *Zuo Commentary* recorded the Chinese history from 722–464 B.C.

[35] *Lv's Spring and Autumn Annals* (*Lv Shi Chunqiu*) was edited at the end of the Warring States Period (475–221 B.C.)when the trend of unification came into being. Being different from the style of the contending among hundred schools of thoughts, the academic style of

the book changed. It was a book of the eclectics which absorbed all kinds of thoughts of the times.

[36] *A Collection of 52 Prescriptions (Wu Shi Er Bing Fang)* is the existing earliest classic on prescription. It was a silk medical book excavated from Han tombs in Mawangdui in Changsha, Hunan province in 1973. The book was named for its record about 52 prescriptions.

[37] Mawangdui is an archaeological site located in Changsha, China. The site consists of two saddle-shaped hills and contained the tombs of three people from the western Han dynasty. The tombs belonged to the first Marquis of Dai, his wife, and a male who is believed to be their son. The site was excavated from 1972 to 1974. Most of the artifacts from Mawangdui are displayed at the Hunan Provincial Museum.

[38] *On Balance (Lun Heng)* is an ancient Chinese philosophical work on materialism by Wang Chong (27–97) in 86 A.D.

[39] Ancient Chinese philosophers believed that the function of the heart was to think, which can be manifested by Chinese characters concerning thinking, such as "思 (thinking)," "想 (thinking)," "念 (miss)," "忘 (forget)," etc. with "心 (the heart)" as their residence. The view has been proved wrong by the modern science.

[40] *Yi Zhuan* is a treatise in Warring States Period (475–221 B.C.) on *A Book of Changes* (a philosophical work concerning the heaven-earth relation, the logical correlations between the hexagrams, lines and remarks affiliated to them, etc.), which was believed to be composed by the King of Wen in the Zhou dynasty (1046–256 B.C.).

[41] *Hsun Tzu (Xun Zi)* is a philosophical work in ancient China. Hsun Tzu (about 313–about 238 B.C.) is one of the great ancient philosophers, litterateurs, political theorists, and Confucian philosophers. Confucius's philosophy focuses on "humanity," Mencius' on "righteousness" and Hsun Tzu's "rites" to regulate people's behaviors.

[42] *Guan Zi*, a philosophical treatise in Spring and Autumn Period (770–476 B.C.), was composed by politician and ideologist Guan Zhong (725–645 B.C.). The treatise was accomplished in about 475–221 B.C. His spirit-qi theory has shed light on China's materialism. His viewpoint of life and his theories about y*in-yang* and Five Elements were widely applied in ancient Chinese medicine.

[43] *Ge Zhi Yu Lun* is a medical treatise by Zhu Zhenheng (1281–1358) in the Yuan dynasty (581–1368 A.D.). It is composed of 42 chapters covering varied medical branches.

[44] *Principles of Correct Diet (Yin Shan Zheng Yao)* was composed by Mongolian nutritionist and medical specialist Hu Sihui, a doctor of the Yuan dynasty's royal court. His viewpoints of health maintenance concerning food and drink cohere with today's requirements of medicine, regimen, nutriology, and hygiene, and still have certain academic and practical values.

[45] *Xi Yuan Lu* is a well-known book on forensic medicine in the Song dynasty by Song Ci (1186–1249, one originator of China's forensic medicine).

[46] Fuxi is a figure talked in the ancient times, who, together with Shennong and Suiren, was called "Three Emperors." It was said that Fuxi was a culture hero reputed to be the inventor of writing, fishing, and trapping.

[47] *Age of Empires (Diwang Shiji)* is a book on Chinese history far from "Three Emperors" (Fuxi, Suiren, and Shennong) to Five August Emperors (Yellow Emperor, Emperor Zhuanxu, Emperor Ku, Emperor Yao, and Emperor Shun), to the emperors of various dynasties till to the Northern Wei Dynasty (386–581).

[48] *Shi Ji Gang Jian* is a historical book.

[49] The oracle bone script (Jia Gu Wen) refers to incised ancient Chinese characters found on oracle bones, which are animal bones or turtle shells used in divination in Bronze Age China.

[50] Yinxu is the ruins of the last capital of China's Shang Dynasty.

[51] Yang Shuda (1885–1956) is an expert in the Chinese language.

[52] *Wuwei Wooden Fragments with the Han Dynasty's Medical Inscription* (*Wuwei Handai Yijian*) was unearthed in Wuwei, Gansu province of China in December 1972. It was believed to be composed before the Eastern Han dynasty (25–200 A.D.), including internal medicine, surgery, prescription, etc.

[53] *Zhi Bai Bing Fang*, a monograph on prescriptions, was unearthed in Wuwei, Gansu province of China in December, 1972. It was believed to be composed before the Eastern Han dynasty, including internal medicine, surgery, prescription, etc.

[54] *Treatise on Febrile Diseases* (*Shanghan Lun*) is one essential part of *Treatise on Exogenous Febrile Disease and Miscellaneous Disease*, mostly concerning exogenous febrile diseases. *Shanghan Lun* is the first classical book in TCM which deals with mechanism, therapeutic principles and methods, prescriptions and herbs.

[55] Yang Shangshan (585–670) was a famous physician of the Sui and Tang dynasties. He served as the royal doctor during the reign of Daye (605–616) and enjoyed a high reputation. He was considered as the first physician to annotate *The Classic of Internal Medicine*.

[56] Wang Bing (about 710–804) was a well-known physician of the Tang dynasty. He was good at medicine and health maintenance. He spent twelve years in systematizing and annotating *Plain Questions*.

[57] Wang Shuhe (201–280) was a well-known physician of the Western Jin dynasty (265–316). He was accomplished in sphygmology and compiled *The Pulse Classic* in 10 volumes according to the experiences summed up by the predecessors and his own clinical experiences. He also reorganized *Treatise on Febrile Diseases*.

[58] *The Essential Remedies* (*Qian Jin Yao Fang*) is a comprehensive clinical classic, composed by Sun Simiao (581–682, the famous physician in the Tang dynasty) in 652.

[59] Chao Yuanfang (550?–630?) was an influential physician in the Sui dynasty (581–618 A.D.). He was a doctor in a royal hospital, taking charge of the compiling of *The General Treatise on the Etiology and Symptomatology of Diseases*.

[60] *Yu Han Fang* is a medical formulary written by Ge Fang in Dynasties of Wei, Jin, North & South.

[61] Ge Hong (283–363) was a Taoist and a famous physician in the Jin dynasty. He was good at alchemy, and his alchemy had a great influence upon the development of chemical and pharmaceutic work. *A Handbook of Prescriptions for Emergencies* is his work.

[62] *Jotting Prescriptions* (*Xiao Pin Fang*) is composed by Chen Yanzhi of the Eastern Jin dynasty (317–420) in about 454–473.

[63] *The Supplement Remedies* (*Qian Jin Yi Fang*) is a supplement to *The Essential Remedies* by Sun Simiao himself in 682.

[64] *A Collection of Effective Recipes* (*Ji Yan Fang*) is a medical formulary composed by Yao Sengyuan (499–583), a famous physician in the North & South dynasty.

[65] Wang Tao (670–755) was a famous physician in the Tang dynasty. Born in a well-known medical family, he was fond of medicine. He compiled *Medical Secrets of an Official* in 40 volumes, which included all the prescriptions before the Tang dynasty.

[66] Cheng Wuji (1066?–1156?) was a noted physician in the Song dynasty. He made an elaborate study of *Treatise on Febrile Diseases*, which had a great influence on the development of the theory on febrile diseases.

[67] All the works in this paragraph are the annotation of Zhang Zhongjing's *Treatise on Febrile Diseases*.

[68] *Classified Canon* (*Lei Jing*) is the classification and annotation of *The Classic of Internal Medicine* by Zhang Jiebing, a famous physician in late Ming Dynasty.

[69] *Essentials for Four Diagnoses* (*Sizhen Jue Wei*) was a masterpiece on TCM's diagnostics by Lin Zhihan (a famous physician in the Qing Dynasty) in 1723. It is composed of 8 volumes focusing on inspection, auscultation and olfaction, interrogation, and pulse taking and palpation.

[70] *Diagnostic Methods Depending on Tongue Inspection* (*Ling Zheng Yan She Fa*) is a TCM dictionary on tongue inspection by Yang Yunfeng in the Qing Dynasty.

[71] *Valuable Prescriptions for Emergency* (*Bei Ji Qian Jin Yaofang*) is highly regarded as China's earliest clinical encyclopedia by Sun Simiao (581–682) in 652.

[72] *A New Book on Health Preservation for Old People* (*Shou Qin Yang Lao Xin Shu*) is China's earliest work on health preservation for old people composed by Chen Zhi in the Song dynasty and supplemented by Zou Xuan in the Yuan dynasty. It covers dietotherapy, medical therapy, and psychotherapy.

[73] *A Book on Health Preserving* (*Yangsheng Lei Zuan*) was a book about health maintenance written by Zhou Shouzhong in the Southern Song dynasty (1127–1279).

[74] *A Book of Changes* (*Yi Jing*) is one of the oldest of the Chinese classic texts. The book centers on the ideas of the dynamic balance of opposites, the evolution of events as a process, and the acceptance of the inevitability of change.

[75] *On Leud States* (*Guo Yu*) is China's earliest historical book on various leud states in the early Spring and Autumn Period: Zhou, Lu, Qi, Jin, Zheng, Chu, Wu and Yue states from 947 B.C. to 453 B.C. Its author is controversial. Many historians such as Si Maqian and Ban Gu believed that its author was Zuo Qiuming.

[76] *Chuang-tzu* (*Zhuang Zi*) is one Taoist classic in allegory. It is composed of three parts. The first part includes 7 chapters, believed to be written by Chuang-tzu himself; the second part includes 15 chapters, believed to be written by his students alone or their cooperation; and the last part including 11 chapters is finished by the later scholars.

[77] *He Guan Zi* is written by Chu's He Guanzi, expounding the academic thoughts of *Yin-yang* School and Taoism in the Warring States Period.

[78] *A Record of Art and Culture, History of the Han Dynasty* (*Han Shu · Yi Wen Zhi*) is the existing earliest historical catalogue literature, written by Ban Gu.

[79] "Taijitu" is an exposition on *Taiji* written by Zhou Dunyi in the Song dynasty. Within 249 words, the essay conveys the Taoist view that *Taiji* is the source of the nature for everything is the result of *yin-yang* interaction and the function of Five Elements.

[80] *An Expounding of the Formularies of the Bureau of the People's Welfare Pharmacies* (*Ju Fang Fahui*) was composed by Zhu Zhenheng in the Yuan dynasty (581–1368 A.D.). The book adopts the question-answer style to make comments on more than 30 issues in *Prescriptions of People's Welfare Pharmacy* (*Taiping Hui Min He Ji Ju Fang*) of the Song dynasty (960–1279 A.D.).

[81] *Yi Guan Bian · Yinyang Lun* was written by Xu Dachun in the Qing dynasty on *yin* and *yang*.

[82] *Diagram Annotation of Classified Canon* (*Lei Jing Tu Yi*), as its name suggests, is the annotation and interpretation of *Classified Canon* (*Lei Jing*) by Zhang Jiebing himself.

[83] *Shang Shu* which consists of 58 chapters is a compilation of documentary records related to events in ancient history of China. Its author is controversial. It is believed that the book was compiled by Confucius and the later Confucians.

[84] *Clinical Experiences of Zhu Danxi* (*Danxi Xinfa*) is a comprehensive medical work by Zhu Zhenheng (his another name is Zhu Danxi) in the Yuan Dynasty.

[85] *Insight from Medical Study* (*Yixue Xinwu*) is a comprehensive medical work by Cheng Zhonglin in 1732.

[86] *Wenbing Tiao Bian* is one of the masterpieces on epidemic disease in China by Wu Tang in 1798.

Glossary

Auscultation and Olfaction (wén zhěn) One of the four diagnostic methods in TCM, consisting of listening and smelling to accord with the dual meanings of the Chinese character. The doctor ascertains the clinic status by listening to abnormal voices and sounds from the patients and by smelling odor of the diseased body.

Baihu Tang (bǎi hǔ tāng) (White Tiger Decoction) A prescription from the *Treatise on Febrile Diseases*. Composition: *Gypsum Fibrosum, Rhizoma Anemarrhenae, Radix Glycyrrhizae Praeparatae*, and *Semen Oryzae Sativae*. Actions: clearing away heat and promoting the production of the residue. Clinical Application: *yangming* disease.

Branches of Twelve Meridians (shí èr jīng bié) The important branches of twelve meridians that enter the body cavity or pass up to the head.

Chaihu Tang (chái hú tāng) (Decoction of *Bupleurum*) A prescription from the *Treatise on Febrile Diseases*. Composition: *Radix Bupleuri, Radix Scutellariae, Radix Gingseng, Radix Glycyrrhizae Praeparatae, Rhizoma Pinelliae, Rhizoma Zingiberis Recens*, and *Fructus Ziziphi Jujubae*. Actions: treating *shaoyang* disease by mediation. Clinical Application: *shaoyang* disease.

Couli (còu lǐ) A term in TCM, refers to the natural texture of the skin and muscles and the spaces between the skin and muscles. It serves as an entrance and outlet for the flow of *qi* and blood and one of the routes for the excretion of body fluids, and has the function of fighting against exogenous pathogenic factors.

Cun Guan Chi (cùn guān chǐ) A collective term for the three places on the wrist over the radial artery where the pulse is felt. *Guan* is located at the radial styloid process, *Cun* is adjacent to it on the distal side, and *Chi* is on the proximal side. The three places of *Cun, Guan*, and *Chi* are respectively known as *Cun*-pulse, *Guan*-pulse, and *Chi*-pulse.

Da Qinglong Tang (dà qīng lóng tāng) (Blue Dragon Decoction) A prescription from the *Treatise on Febrile Diseases*. Composition: *Herba Ephedrae, Ramulus Cinnamoni, Semen Armeniaccae Amarum, Radix Glycyrrhizae Praeparatae, Rhizoma Zingiberis Recens, Fructus Ziziphi Jujubae*, and *Gypsum Fibrosum*. Actions: relieving exterior syndrome by means of diaphoresis, clearing away heat and relieving restlessness. Clinical Application: exterior-excess syndrome due to exogenous wind with internal heat.

Daoyin Exercise (dǎo yǐn) A term in TCM, refers to a series of breathing exercises practiced by Taoists to cultivate internal energy of the body based upon the principles of TCM. It was an ancient precursor of *qigong*, and was practiced in Chinese Taoist monasteries for health and spiritual cultivation.

Defensive *Qi* (wèi qì) A kind of *yang-qi* which originates from food. It moves out of the meridians and collaterals, and has the functions of protecting the human body against exogenous pathogenic factors.

Disease-cause Syndrome Differentiation (bìng yīn biàn zhèng) The analysis and differentiation of pathological conditions attributable to different kinds of causal factors for making a diagnosis.

Eight Extra Meridians (qí jīng bā mài) A general term for the *Du, Ren, Chong, Dai, Yinqiao, Yangqiao, Yinwei,* and *Yangwei* meridians, which have no direct relationship with any of the *zang-fu* organs or exterior-interior coordination between them and they are different from the twelve meridians. Their functions are strengthening the ties between the meridians and regulating the *qi* and blood inside the twelve regular meridians.

Eight-principle Syndrome Differentiation (bā gāng biàn zhèng) The process of diagnosing a syndrome by analyzing the patient's condition according to the eight principles, i.e., differentiating the location of a disease between exterior and interior, distinguishing the nature of a disease between cold and heat, identifying the patient's condition as deficiency or excess, and generalizing the syndrome or pattern as *yin* or *yang*.

Essential *Qi* (jīng qì) A general reference to the refined substance and its functions, such as reproductive essence and nutrient *qi* derived from food essence.

Exhaustion of *Ying* (tuō yíng) A disease in TCM. 1. It refers to the consumptive disease due to impairment by emotional stress. It is marked by vexation in mind, chest pain and asthenia, perspiration and palpitation, restlessness, lassitude and anorexia. It is treated by regulating *qi* by alleviation of mental depression. 2. It refers to edema syndrome due to emotional depression. It is marked by slight swelling in the initial stage without changes in skin color while exacerbation by years with edema hardlike stone, etc. It is advisable to treat the said disease by regulating *qi* and subduing swelling and edema.

Fifteen Main Collaterals (shí wǔ luò, or shí wǔ luò mài, or shí wǔ bié luò) Each of the fourteen meridians has a main collateral–together with the great collateral of the spleen, there are fifteen in all–which communicate with the exterior and interior of the body.

Five Fauna-mimic Frolics (wǔ qín xì) A kind of gymnastics invented by Hua Tuo in the Eastern Han dynasty (25–220 A.D.), which imitates the movements of such five types of wildlife as tiger, deer, bear, ape, and bird.

Five Emotions (wǔ zhì) A collective term for joy, anger, anxiety, grief and fear, which may turn into fire if in excess.

Five Notes (wǔ yīn) A term referring to such five notes as jué, zhǐ, gōng, shāng and yǔ, which respectively mate five *zang*-organs, i.e., jué corresponding to the livers, zhǐ to the heart, gōng to the spleen, shāng to lungs and yǔ to kidneys. From *Spiritual Pivot,* Chapter 71.

Five Smells (wǔ xiù) A term referring to such five smells as foul, empyreumatic, fragrant, fishy, and rancid, which respectively correspond to five *zang*-organs, i.e., foul corresponding to the liver, empyreumatic to the heart, fragrant to the spleen, fishy to lungs and rancid to kidneys. From *Plain Questions,* Chapter 9.

Five Sounds (wǔ shēng) A term referring to such five sounds as shout, laugh, sing, cry and groan which are related to five *zang*-organs, i.e., shout is connected with the liver, laugh with the heart, sing with the spleen, cry with the lungs, and groan with the kidneys. From *Plain Questions,* Chapter 5.

Fuliang (fú liáng) An ancient name for a disease with epigastria fullness and mass, mostly due to stagnation of *qi* and blood.

Gegen Tang (gě gēn tāng) (Decoction of *Radix Puerariae*) A prescription from the

Treatise on Febrile Diseases. Composition: *Radix Puerariae, Herba Ephedrae, Ramulus Cinnamoni, Radix Paeoniae, Radix Glycyrrhizae Praeparatae, Rhizoma Zingiberis Recens*, and *Fructus Ziziphi Jujubae*. Actions: relieving exterior syndrome by means of diaphoresis. Clinical Application: exterior syndrome due to exogenous wind-cold.

Guizhi Jia Fuzi Tang (guì zhī jiā fù zī tāng) (Decoction of Cassia Twig plus Monkshood) A prescription the from *Treatise on Febrile Diseases*. Composition: *Ramulus Cinnamoni*, and *Radix Paeoniae*, and *Radix Glycyrrhizae Praeparatae, Rhizoma Zingiberis Recens, Fructus Ziziphi Jujubae*, and *Radix Aconiti Lateralis Praeparata*. Actions: warming up *yang* for repelling exogenous pathogenic factors. Clinical Application: *taiyang* disease marked by continuous perspiration, aversion to wind and difficult urination.

Guizhi Tang (guì zhī tāng) (Decoction of Cassia Twig) A prescription from the *Treatise on Febrile Diseases*. Composition: *Ramulus Cinnamoni, Radix Paeoniae, Radix Glycyrrhizae Praeparatae, Rhizoma Zingiberis Recens*, and *Fructus Ziziphi Jujubae*. Actions: expelling pathogenic factors from the muscles and skin, and regulating nutrient *qi* and defensive *qi* to relieve exterior syndrome. Clinical Application: wind-attack syndrome of *taiyang* disease.

He-Sea Acupoint (hé xué) A term in TCM referring to one of the five-shu acupoints. There is one He-Sea acupoint in each of the twelve meridians, situated near elbows or knees where meridian *qi* gathers from the end of the extremes, just like the confluence of streams with the most exuberant meridian *qi* there.

Inspection (wàng zhěn) One of the four diagnostic methods. It is a diagnostic technique to examine a man's body by using the eyes, including inspection of vitality, complexion, expression, behavior, body surface, tongue, excreta, secretions, etc.

Interrogation (wèn zhěn) One of four techniques of diagnosis. It is a diagnostic technique for the doctor to inquire of the patient or his companion about the onset, progress, course of treatment, present symptoms, past history of the illness, and other conditions related to the illness.

Jing-River Acupoint (jīng xué) A term in TCM referring to one of the five-shu acupoints. It means that meridian *qi* in this acupoint blooms like a river. Twelve meridians each have their own Jing-River acupoints, which are located in the forearms or the crura.

Jing-Well Acupoint (jīng xué) A term in TCM referring to one of the five-shu acupoints. It means that meridian *qi* is very tiny in this acupoint just like a well oozing out at first and it is called "Jing," which means "Well." Twelve meridians each have their own Jing-Well acupoints, which are at the end of four limbs.

Jiuzhen (jiǔ zhēn) Nine needles used in acupuncture in ancient China, i.e., sagittal needle, ovoid-tip needle, blunt needle, ensiform needle, sword-shaped needle, round-shaped needle, filiform needle, long needle, and large needle.

Life Gate (mìng mén) A term in TCM, taking the house of water and fire as the root of life, closely related to kidneys both physiologically and pathologically. The genuine fire in the life gate, i.e., *life gate* fire, refers to kidney fire, and the genuine water in the *life gate* refers to kidney *yin*.

Mahuang Fuzi Xixin Tang (má huáng fù zī xì xīn tāng) (Decoction of Ephedra, Monkshood and Asarum) A prescription from the *Treatise on Febrile Diseases*. Composition:

Herba Ephedrae, *Radix Aconiti Lateralis Praeparata*, and *Herba Asari*. Actions: warming up the meridians and nourishing *yang*, inducing diaphoresis to dispel cold. Clinical Application: cold syndrome due to *yang* deficiency.

Mahuang Tang (má huáng tāng) (Ephedra Decoction) A prescription from the *Treatise on Febrile Diseases*. Composition: *Herba Ephedrae, Ramulus Cinnamoni, Semen Armeniaccae Amarum*, and *Radix Glycyrrhizae Praeparatae*. Actions: inducing diaphoresis and relieving asthma. Clinical Application: exterior-excess syndrome due to exogenous wind-cold.

Nutrient *Qi* (yíng qì) The essential substance circulating in the blood vessels, meridians and collaterals. It is derived from food and drink which are transformed and transported by the spleen and stomach, and has the functions of nourishing all parts of the body.

Pulse Taking and Palpation (qiè zhěn) One of the four diagnostic methods. It consists of pulse feeling and palpation. The pulse feeling is to feel the pulse and the palpation is to touch, feel, press and weigh down a certain part of the disease and to diagnose diseases combined with other methods (inspection, auscultation and olfaction, and interrogation).

***Qi* (qì)** A term referring to the vital substances comprising the human body and maintaining its life activities, such as the *qi* of water and food essence, the air of breathing, etc.

***Qi jiao* (qì jiāo)** A TCM term referring to the convergence of descending celestial *qi* and ascending terrestrial *qi*, which is believed the source of the generation, change, and transformation of *yin-yang* and all things.

Qiqing (qī qíng) A term referring to the seven actions as to combine different Chinese medicinal herbs according to the needs of the disease, i.e., single effect, mutual reinforcement, mutual assistant, mutual restraint, mutual detoxication, mutual inhibition, and incompatibility.

Seven Emotions (qī qíng) A general term for seven kinds of excessive emotions, i.e., terror, anger, anxiety, contemplation, grief, fear, and joy, which can cause the dysfunction of vital energy.

Shu-Stream Acupoint (shū xué) A term in TCM referring to one of the five-shu acupoints. Twelve meridians each have their own Shu-Stream acupoints, which are situated in the wrists or the metatarsal joints where meridian *qi* is so powerful that it pours into the depth like a stream, and thus it gets its name.

Sini Tang (sì nì tāng) (Decoction for Resuscitation) A prescription from the *Treatise on Febrile Diseases*. Composition: *Radix Aconiti Praeparatae, Rhizoma Zingiberis*, and *Radix Glycyrrhizae Praeparatae*. Actions: Recuperating depleted *yang* to rescue the patient from collapse. Clinical Application: syndrome of hyperactivity of *yin* due to *yang* exhaustion.

Six Excesses (liù yín) A collective term for pathogenic factors, i.e., wind, cold, summer-heat, dampness, dryness, and heat either exogenous or endogenous, which, if they are excessive or occur untimely, will cause illness.

Six Meridians (liù jīng) A collective term for *taiyang* meridian, *yangming* meridian, *shaoyang* meridian, *taiyin* meridian, *shaoyin* meirian, and *jueyin* meiridian, which, in conformity with the twelve meridians, may be subdivided into the six meridians of the hand and the six meridians of the foot.

Tendons of Twelve Meridians (shí èr jīng jīn) The joints of the system of meridians and collaterals on the surface of the human body. As their distribution is closely related to the tendons and muscles, they are known as the tendons. The pathological changes in the tendons of twelve meridians are mostly manifested as relaxation, contraction, stiffening and convulsion.

Theory of Meridians (jīng luò xué shuō) An important component of traditional Chinese medical theory, according to which there exists within the human body a system of conduits through which *qi* and blood circulate, and by which the internal organs are connected with the superficial organs and tissues, and the body is made of an organic whole.

Thoracic Obstruction (xiōng bì) A morbid condition due to turbid phlegm or blood stasis caused by failure of *yang-qi* in the chest to disperse, marked by choking pain and fullness in the chest, and asthmatic breathing with the inability to lie flat.

Tiangui (tiān guǐ) A term in TCM, refers to the substance that can promote human growth, development, and reproductive function, and that can maintain women's regular menstruation and normal pregnancy. It originates from the kidney essence, and gradually becomes abundant with the nourishment of the acquired food.

Triple Energizer (sān jiāo) A collective term for the three portions of the body cavity, through which *qi* and fluids are transmitted. "Upper energizer" refers to the portion above the diaphragm housing the heart and lungs; "middle energizer" refers to the portion between the diaphragm and the umbilicus housing the spleen and stomach; "lower energizer" refers to the portion below the umbilicus cavity housing the kidneys, bladder, small and large intestines, and includes the liver owing to its pathophysiologic relation to the kidneys.

Twelve Cutaneous Regions (shí èr pí bù) The regions of the skin reflecting the functioning of the twelve regular meridians respectively.

Twelve Meridians (shí èr jīng) It is also known as the regular meridians. They are the lung meridian of hand *taiyin* (LU), the large intestine meridian of hand *yangming* (LI), the stomach meridian of foot *yangming* (ST), the spleen meridian of foot *taiyin* (SP), the heart meridian of hand *shaoyin* (HT), the small intestine meridian of hand *taiyang* (SI), the bladder meridian of foot *taiyang* (BL), the kidney meridian of foot *shaoyin* (KI), the pericardium meridian of hand *jueyin* (PC), the *triple energizer* meridian of hand *shaoyang* (TE), the gallbladder meridian of foot shaoyang (GB), and the liver meridian of foot *jueyin* (LR). They are the main passages of *qi* and blood.

Weijing Tang (wěi jìng tāng) (Reed Stem Decoction) A prescription from *The Essential Remedies*. Composition: *Rhizoma Phragmitis*, and *Semen Coicis*, *Semen Benincasae*, and *Semen Persicae*. Actions: clearing away heat from the lung and resolving phlegm, removing stasis and promoting pus discharge. Clinical Application: pulmonary abscess.

Wu Lin San (wǔ líng sǎn) (Powder of Five Drugs Containing Poria) A prescription from the *Treatise on Febrile Diseases*. Composition: *Polyporus*, *Rhizoma Alismatis*, *Rhizoma Atractylodis*, *Poria*, and *Ramulus Cinnamomi*. Actions: inducing diuresis, eliminating dampness, warming *yang*, and promoting *qi* function.

Xianghuo (xiàng huǒ) A term referring to a kind of physiological fire. It can warm and nourish the viscera and promote their functional activities. It originates from *life gate* and is stored in the liver, gallbladder, and *triple energizer*.

***Yang* (yáng)** A term referring to the active, masculine cosmic principle in Chinese dualistic philosophy.

***Yin* (yīn)** A term referring to the passive, female cosmic principle in Chinese dualistic philosophy.

Ying (yíng) (also called Nutrient *Qi* (yíng qì)) A term in TCM referring to the essential substance circulating in the channels and blood vessels. It comes from food essence transformed and transported by the spleen and stomach so far as the formation is concerned. It originates from *middle-energizer* (the portion between the diaphragm and the umbilicus housing the spleen and stomach), and has two functions: One is to produce blood and the other is to nourish the whole body.

Ying-Spring Acupoint (yíng xué) A term in TCM referring to one of the five-shu acupoints. It means that meridian *qi* gradually increases in this acupoint just like a spring. Twelve meridians each have their own Ying-Spring acupoints, which are located in the metacarpophalangeal or metatarsophalangeal joints.

***Zang-fu* Organs (zàng fǔ)** A collective term for all internal organs, including *zang* organs, *fu* organs, and extra *fu* organs. *Zang* organs refer to the internal organs that produce, transform, and store essential *qi*. Specifically, they are the heart, the liver, the spleen, lungs, and kidneys. *Fu* organs refer to the internal organs that receive, contain, and transmit food and drink. Specifically, *fu* organs are the gallbladder, stomach, large intestine, small intestine, urinary bladder, and *triple energizer*, all related to food digestion and fluid transmission. Extra *fu* organs refer to the brain, spinal cord, bones, blood vessels, gallbladder, and uterus.

***Zang-fu* Organs Syndrome Differentiation (zàng fǔ biàn zhèng)** The differentiation of syndromes or the identification of patterns according to the pathological changes of *zang-fu* organs.

***Zang-xiang* (zàng xiàng)** *Zang* collectively refers to the internal viscera and tissues, as well as their functions and changes, which cannot be directly observed by eyes. On the contrary, *xiang* refers to those observable external organs and tissues, as well as their functions and changes. *Zang-xiang* as a term refers to the visceral manifestation, namely, the outward manifestations of the internal organs through which physiological functions as well as their pathological changes can be detected and the state of health judged.

Zhuling Tang (zhū líng tāng) (Umbellate Pore Decoction) A prescription, from the *Treatise on Febrile Diseases*. Composition: *Polyporus, Rhizoma Alismatis, Poria, Colla Corri Asini* (melted), and *Talcum*. Actions: nourishing *yin*, clearing away heat, and promoting urination. Clinical Application: *yin* impairment by retention of water and heat.

Xiao Chengqi Tang (xiāo chéng qì tāng) (Decoction for Purgation) A prescription from the *Treatise on Febrile Diseases*. Composition: *Radix et Rhizoma Rhei, Cortex Magnoliae Officinalis*, and *Radix Glycyrrhizae Praeparatae*. Actions: clearing away heat and relieving constipation. Clinical Application: excessive-heat syndrome of *Yangming* meridian.

Subject Index

Academic System, 1
acumoxibustion, 6
Acupoint Selection, 97
Acupuncture, 1, 76, 97, 111
analogy, 79, 104, 105
asthenia, 4, 30, 72
asthenia syndrome, 30, 72
Auscultation and Olfaction, 4, 94, 124
Behcet's disease, 52
bio-psycho-social-medical model, 101
blood phase, 8, 14, 36
child organ affecting mother organ, 91, 92
child-mother transmission, 91
Clinical System, 4, 26
cold, 2, 29, 36, 77
cold syndrome, 34, 51, 73
cold syndrome with pseudo-heat symptoms, 73
compound-symptom-and-prescription-based, 28
Contradictions, 3
contradictory unities, 47
cooling therapy, 4, 33, 107
correspondence between man and nature, 3, 9, 43
Counterevidence, 106
clinical achievements, 23
Counterrestraint, 83, 87, 93
damp-heat diseases, 49
Daoyin exercise 24, 121
Decoction, 2, 31, 33
defensive phase, 8, 14, 36
defensive *qi*, 59, 123
deficiency-cold syndrome, 48
deficiency-heat syndrome, 48
deficient earth being overrestrained by wood, 92
depletion of essence, 46
dialectical approach, 104
diaphoresis, 4, 32, 107
diet therapy, 23, 34
disease, 27, 29, 31, 49
disease differentiation, 31, 53
disease-differentiation-based treatment, 47
drug-symptom, 32
earth, 20, 80, 83, 90
emesis, 4, 33, 107
environmental-health-medical model, 101

environment-body-mind medical model, 102, 103
epidemic diseases, 45, 107
epidemic febrile diseases, 49
Essence, 19, 42
Essence-*Qi*-Spirit Theory, 19
evil *qi*, 21, 59
excess, 4, 36, 60
excess-cold syndrome, 48
excess syndrome, 35
excessive-heat syndrome, 48
exhaustion of ying, 46, 122
exogenous febrile diseases, 4, 33
exogenous pathogenic factors, 29, 72
exterior, 4, 48
exterior syndrome, 32, 48, 123
extreme *yang* like *yin*, 73
extreme *yin* like *yang*, 73
exuberant *yang* repelling *yin*, 73
fire, 20, 80, 83, 90
five constituents, 21, 39, 90
Five Elements, 20, 79
five emotions, 21, 97
five fauna-mimic frolics, 13, 122
five flavors, 30, 77
five materials, 20, 78
five sense organs, 21, 90
five tastes, 43
forensic medicine, 23
four properties, 30, 76
fu-organs, 39, 69, 90
Gegen Tang, 31, 122
giving prevention the priority, 3
Guizhi Jia Fuzi Tang, 32, 125
Guizhi Tang, 32, 123
healthy *qi*, 23, 59
heat, 4, 29, 36, 77
heat syndrome with pseudo-cold symptoms, 73
heat syndrome, 35, 49, 71, 72
Heuristic Method, 105
Holism, 3, 18, 38
holistic approach, 104
impairment of *yin* involving *yang*, 65, 72
Inspection, 4, 94, 123
interior, 4, 48
interior syndrome, 67, 71

Interpromotion, 83, 89, 95
Interpromotion Transmission, 91
Interrestraint, 84, 89, 92
Interrogation, 4, 94, 124
Judging the Interior from the Exterior Manifestations, 40
Jueyin disease, 31
knife-like needle, 2
Lao-tzu, 57
life gate, 30, 125
lung-*qi*, 47, 97
lung-*yin*, 47, 96
Mafei San, 6, 23
Mahuang Fuzi Xixin Tang, 32, 123
Massage, 7, 111
medical formulary, 6, 34
medical model, 101–103
medical system, 3
Meridian system, 40
meridian tropism of drugs, 24–25
meridians and collaterals, 3, 69
metal, 20, 80, 83, 90
miscellaneous diseases, 4, 33
monism of *qi*, 9, 55
mother-child transmission, 91
moxibustion, 2, 111
mutual promotion between metal and water, 96
mutual-rejection between *yin* and *yang*, 73
non-drug therapies,
"nourishing *yin*" school, 103
nutrient phase, 8, 14, 36
nutrient *qi*, 59, 126
Overrestrain, 86, 92
pathological outlook, 12
pharmacology, 5, 7, 8
philosophical methodology, 99
physiological outlook, 11
predominant *yin* rejecting *yang*, 73
Prescription, 2, 4, 112
prescription-syndrome, 32–33
psychic-medical model, 99
psychotherapies, 103
pulse conditions, 6, 32, 94
Pulse differentiation, 6
Pulse Taking and Palpation, 4, 94, 124
purgation, 4, 33, 77, 107
"purgation" school, 103
Qi, 9, 19, 126
qi activity, 59
qi deficiency, 41, 66
qi jiao, 43, 124
qi phase, 8, 14, 36
qigong, 51
qiqing, 30, 124

qi-transformation, 63, 70
regulating therapy, 4, 33, 107
relative deficiency of *yin* or *yang*, 74, 76
relative predominance of *yin* or *yang*, 74, 75
resolving therapy, 4, 33
Shaoyang disease, 31, 121
Shaoyin disease, 31
shu xie, 39, 92
single-symptom-and-single-medicine-based practice, 28
Sini Tang, 31, 124
six excesses, 21, 124
six kinds of *qi*, 18, 60
Six Meridians, 4, 124
Speculating the Interior from the Exterior, 108
Spirit, 10, 19
"spleen-invigorating" school, 102
stone-needle practice, 1
superficiality and origin, 50
supplementing, 4, 33, 107
symptom, 48
Syndrome, 12, 31, 49
syndrome differentiation, 49–52
system approach, 104
Taijitu, 68
Taiyang disease, 31, 123
Taiyin disease, 31
Tao, 57, 60, 68
Taoism, 17, 57
TCM's general philosophical methods, 103
TCM's therapeutic outlook, 14
temporal transmission, 91, 93
The Architecture of TCM, 107
The Cold School of Medicine, 4
the different diseases with the same syndrome, 52
the disorder of mother organ involving child organ, 30
the eight diagnostic principles, 4
the exterior wind-cold syndrome, 50
the exterior wind-heat syndrome, 50
the external excess syndrome, 50
the four diagnostic methods, 4, 47
the law of pathogenesis, 41
The Method of Insight, 107
the movement of *qi*, 58
the observation of complexion, 41
The oracle bone script, 27, 60, 77, 118
the primordial *qi*, 9, 57
the principles of TSD, 36, 51
the relativity of *yin-yang*, 62
the same disease with different syndromes, 31, 52

Subject Index

The School for Strengthening the Spleen and Stomach, 4
"the school of cold and cool," 103
the universality of *yin-yang*, 62
The Yin-Nourishing School, 4
therapeutic methods, 4, 97
therapeutic principles, 51, 53, 77
to enrich earth to generate mental,
to enrich water to nourish wood, 96
to focus on the principal cause of diseases, 13
to inhibit wood and support earth, 97
to purge fire and supplement water, 97
to purge the child organ, 96
to regulate *yin* and *yang*, 13, 75
to reinforce metal to inhibit wood, 97
to reinforce the mother organ, 96
to strengthen vital energy to eliminate pathogenic factors, 13
to supplement fire to reinforce earth, 96
tongue observation, 41
Traditional Chinese Medicine, 1, 110–113
Transformation of Interrestraint, 92
treating cold syndrome with warm therapy, 49
treating disease before its onset, 3, 13
treating excess syndrome with purgation, 75
treating heat syndrome with cold therapy, 75
treating the same disease with different methods, 47
treating *yang* disease from *yin* aspect, 76
treating *yin* disease from *yang* aspect, 76
triple energizer, 5, 126
TSD, 47, 51, 54
Twelve Meridians, 39, 76, 126

waning of both *yin* and *yang*, 66
warming therapy, 4, 33, 107
water, 20, 81, 83, 90
waxing of both *yin* and *yang*, 66
wood, 20, 80, 83, 89
wood overrestraining earth, 85, 92
xianghuo, 36, 125
yang impairment affecting *yin*, 72
yang meridians, 42, 48, 76
yang syndrome, 35, 67, 75
yang waning and *yin* waxing, 66
yang, 62–63, 126
Yangming disease, 31, 121
yang-qi, 57, 68, 75
yin syndrome, 35, 67, 75
yin waning and *yang* waxing, 66
yin, 62–63, 126
yin-fluid, 48, 75
yin-qi, 57, 68, 71
yin-yang balance, 12, 66
yin-yang imbalance, 12, 73, 75
Yin-yang Interaction, 63
Yin-yang Interdependence, 66–69
yin-yang mutual impairment, 72
Yin-yang Opposition, 65–66
yin-yang theory, 60–67
Yin-yang Transformation, 68–69
Yin-yang Wane-wax, 67–68
Yin-yang, 19, 62–63
zang-fu organs, 11, 126
zang-organs, 40, 69, 91
zang-xiang theory, 11, 40, 105
Zhuling Tang, 31, 126

Title Index

A Book of Changes, 56, 60, 120
A Book on Health Preserving, 45, 120
A Collection of Effective Recipes, 34, 119
A Collection of 52 Prescriptions, 17, 118
A Handbook of Prescriptions for
    Emergencies, 7, 119
A New Book on Health Preservation for Old
    People, 45, 120
Acumoxibustion on Mingtang
    Acupoint, 6, 116
Age of Empires, 27, 118
An Expounding of the Formularies of the
    Bureau of the People's Welfare Phar-
    macies, 62, 120
Chiseling Open the Regularity of Qian
    (Heaven), 9, 117
Chuang-tzu, 56, 120
Classified Canon, 40, 120
Clinical Experiences of Zhu
    Danxi, 107, 120
Compendium of Materia Medica, 8, 117
Corrections of the Errors in Medical
    Works, 5, 116
Diagram Annotation of Classified
    Canon, 68, 120
Effective Prescriptions Handed Down for
    Generations, 7, 117
Essentials for Four Diagnosis, 41
Ge Zhi Yu Lun, 22, 118
Guan Zi, 20, 118
History of the Later Han Dynasty, 2, 115
Hsun Tzu, 20, 118
Huainan Tzu, 1, 115
Insight from Medical Study, 107, 120
Jotting Prescriptions, 34, 119
Lv's Spring and Autumn Annals, 18, 117
Medical Secrets of an Official, 7, 116
On Balance, 19, 118
On Leud States, 56, 120
Plain Questions, 2, 115
Prescriptions Assigned to the Three Cate
    gories of Pathogenic Factors of
    Diseases, 4, 116
Prescriptions for Midwifery, 7, 117
Principles of Correct Diet, 24, 118

Records of the Historian, 2, 115
Shang Shu, 78, 120
Shi Ji Gang Jian, 27, 118
Six Legal Documents of Tang
    Dynasty, 117
Spiritual Pivot, 10, 117
Synopsis of the Golden Chamber, 12, 117
Taoist Lin's Secret Recipes for Wounds and
    Bone-setting, 7, 116
The A-B Classic of Acumoxibustion, 6, 116
The Book of Songs, 2, 115
The Chinese Materia Medica of the Tang
    Dynasty, 7
The Classic of Acupuncture, 6, 116
The Classic of Internal Medicine, 2, 115
The Classic of Materia Medica, 4, 116
The Classic of Medical Problems, 4, 115
The Classic of Mountains and
    Rivers, 2, 115
The Classified Materia Medica, 8, 117
The Essential Remedies, 33, 119
The General Treatise on the Etiology and
    Symptomatology of Diseases, 4, 116
The Newly Revised Materia Medica, 7
The Pulse Classic, 6, 116
The Supplement Remedies, 34, 119
Therapeusis of Pediatric Diseases, 4, 116
Treatise on Exogenous Febrile Diseases and
    Miscellaneous Diseases, 3, 115
Treatise on Febrile Diseases, 30, 119
Treatise on Infant Health and Pediatric
    Prescriptions, 7, 117
Treatise on Pestilence, 9, 117
Valuable Prescriptions for
    Emergency, 45, 120
Well-tried Formulae by Su and
    Shen, 8
Wenbing Tiao Bian, 107, 120
Wuwei Wooden Fragments with the Han
    Dynasty's Medical Inscription, 29, 119
Xi Yuan Lu, 24, 118
Yu Han Fang, 34, 119
Zhi Bai Bing Fang, 29, 119
Zuo Commentary, 18, 117

Name Index

Bian Que, 23
Chao Yuanfang, 4, 119
Chen Wuze, 4, 36
Chen Yanzhi, 34
Cheng Guopeng, 107
Cheng Wuji, 35, 119
Ge Hong, 34, 119
He Xiu, 56
Hua Tuo, 6, 13, 23
Huangpu Mi, 6
Li Gao, 4, 102
Li Shizhen, 8, 24
Liu Wansu, 4, 35, 103
Liu Xin, 56
Liu Zongyuan, 56
Qian Yi, 4
Shennong, 1, 116
Sun Simiao, 7, 34
Wang Bing, 33, 34, 119
Wang Chong, 56, 118
Wang Fuzhi, 56
Wang Qingren, 5, 116
Wang Shuhe, 6, 33, 119

Wang Tao, 34, 119
Wang Tingxiang, 60
Wei Yilin, 7
Wu Tang, 5, 107, 120
Wu Youke, 5, 9, 107
Xu Shuwei, 35
Xun Kuang, 17
Yang Shangshan, 33, 119
Yao Sengyuan, 34, 119
Ye Gui, 5, 53
Yi He, 56, 60
Yi Yin, 2
Yu Liu, 7, 117
Zhang Congzheng, 4, 36, 103
Zhang Jiebin, 5, 60, 105
Zhang Zai, 56, 60
Zhang Zhongjing, 4, 111
Zhao Xianke, 5
Zhou Dunyi, 60, 120
Zhu Zhenheng, 4, 22, 103
Zhuang Zhou, 56
Zou Yan, 60